CLINICIAN'S
ILLUSTRATED
DICTIONARY OF
GASTROENTEROLOGY

A – C

CLINICIAN'S ILLUSTRATED DICTIONARY OF GASTROENTEROLOGY

Anthony C Smith MBChB MRCP (Lond.)
Department of Gastroenterology, Northwick Park Hospital, UK

Ashley B Price MA BM BCh MRC Path
Department of Pathology, Northwick Park Hospital, UK

A – C

Presented as a service to medicine by Glaxo Laboratories Limited

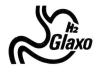

Science Press

Acknowledgements

The authors would like to thank Professor John S. Fordtran
and the W.B. Saunders Company for permission to reproduce
Tables 3, 4, 6 and 7 which originally appeared in *Gastrointestinal
Diseases* third edition 1983, Professor Ian A.D. Bouchier and
Ballière Tindall for permission to reproduce Tables 9, 12 and
14 which originally appeared in *Gastroenterology*, third edition
1982, and the editors of the *American Journal of Surgery* for
permission to reproduce Table 5.

The authors would also like to thank Dr A.J. Levi for Figures 17
and 17b, Dr E. Hudson for Figure 31, Mrs B. Sandin for Figure
34, Miss S. Thom for Figure 38 and Cambmac Instruments for
Figure 46.

The sponsorship of this book does not imply approval or
otherwise of any of the products of the sponsor by the authors.

British Library Cataloguing in Publication Data

Price, Ashley B.
Clinician's Illustrated Dictionary of Gastroenterology

1. Gastroenterology – Dictionaries
I. Title II. Smith, Anthony C
616. 3'3' 00321 RC801

ISBN 1 – 870026 – 15 – 2

Introduction

The Clinician's Illustrated Dictionary of Gastroenterology is a comprehensive reference book of particular use to general practitioners, hospital doctors and their staff. The authors have included tables, figures and illustrations which present additional material in a simple and accessible form. The dictionary is concise but where significant terms require greater detail the definitions have been appropriately extended.

The system of cross references employed in the dictionary has three features. A 'see' reference occurs where a term is more commonly known under a different name. A 'see also' reference passes the reader on to information which is related and supplementary to the definition. Many entries have a number of possible alternative expressions and these appear under their most commonly used term with alternatives mentioned as 'also known as'. The alternative will have its own entry cross referenced to the most commonly used term.

Diseases, signs, syndromes and tests which are known by their proper names are entered under those names. In most cases biographical details have been added.

A C Smith
A B Price

London, 1987

Abbreviations

Abbreviations are usually explained when first introduced within the definition itself but some commonly used abbreviations and their meanings are given here. Shortened forms for such as enzymes, diseases and tests have been avoided throughout the dictionary except where the abbreviation is better known, as in AIDS and DNA.

c   carbon
cm   centimetres
dl   decilitres
DNA   deoxyribonucleic acid
ECG   electrocardiogram
ERCP   endoscopic retrograde
          cholangiopancreatography
ESR   erythrocyte sedimentation rate
gm   gram
gm/l   grams per litre
gm/dl   grams per decilitre
HBe   hepatitis e antigen
HBsAg   hepatitis B surface antigen
kg   kilogram
mequv/l   milliequivalents per litre
mm   millimetre
mmHg   millimetre mercury

A

Abbott-Miller tube
(*also known as* Miller-Abbott tube)
(William Osler Abbott, U.S. physician,
1902-1943; Thomas Grier Miller, U.S.
physician, born 1886) A double lumen tube
used for intestinal decompression.

ABC
see *Aspiration biopsy cytology*

Abdomen
That part of the body cavity between the
chest (thorax) and pelvis. It is lined by a
serous membrane, the peritoneum, which
contains the visceral organs (stomach,
small intestine, colon, liver, gallbladder,
pancreas, spleen).

The abdomen is separated from the
chest by the diaphragm but is continuous
with the pelvis at the pelvic brim. It can be
divided into six regions (Figure 1). Varying
shapes of abdomen are recognized, such as
scaphoid, or boat shaped abdomen, where
the anterior wall is sunken and has a
concave contour.

An *acute abdomen* or *surgical abdomen*
refers to severe abdominal pain, usually of
sudden onset and often is associated with
inflammation, perforation, obstruction,

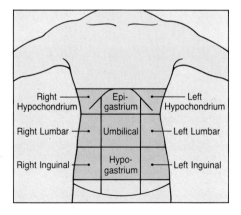

Figure 1 **Abdomen**. Regions of the abdomen.

infarction or rupture of the intra-
abdominal organs. Urgent assessment is
necessary and emergency surgical
intervention is frequently required. Causes
include acute cholecystitis or
appendicitis, perforated peptic ulcer,
strangulated hernia, superior mesenteric
artery thrombosis and splenic rupture.
Other causes of abdominal pain, however,
must be borne in mind, such as urinary
infection, myocardial infarction, porphyria,
and, especially in children, right lower
lobe pneumonia. Urgent assessment and
investigation using plain abdominal and
chest x-rays, blood cultures, serum
electrolytes, amylase, and midstream urine
tests are mandatory. Further tests, such
as ECG, HIDA scans, and abdominal
ultrasound or abdominal paracentesis
may be helpful in some circumstances.
Emergency surgical intervention is often
required.

Abdominal (intestinal) angina
An uncommon condition usually caused
by ischaemia of the gut due to atherosclerosis affecting the major blood
vessels supplying the intestine. Presenting
symptoms are recurrent abdominal pain
occurring 15 to 30 minutes after a meal
and lasting several hours, weight loss, and
an abdominal bruit. Patients are usually
elderly.

Abdominal aorta
That part of the aorta traversing the
abdomen.

Abdominal hernia
see *Hernia*

Abdominal pain
Pain experienced or felt in the abdomen
and often, but not always, due to pathology
from within. The correct interpretation of
abdominal pain is a demanding challenge
of any physician's ability, requiring
experience and judgement. A meticulous
history and physical examination is
extremely important.

Abdominal pain

Mechanisms of abdominal pain include inflammation of the parietal peritoneum, obstruction of a hollow viscus, and vascular disturbance. Pain may be referred to the abdomen from other sites such as thorax, spine or genitalia, and may be attributable to metabolic or neurogenic causes.

Inflammation of the parietal peritoneum is usually of a steady, aching character and localized over the site of inflammation. Gastric acid and pancreatic juice incite very severe pain while blood and urine produce much less pain. The pain of peritoneal inflammation is exacerbated by pressure over the peritoneum.

Obstruction of a hollow viscus leads to intermittent, colicky pain, which may become continuous with occasional exacerbations, when the organ is distended or dilated. The pain from small intestinal obstruction is usually periumbilical and poorly localized. However, sudden distension of the biliary tree produces a constant steady pain, when the term biliary colic becomes misleading.

Vascular disturbance includes embolism or thrombosis of the superior mesenteric artery or dissection of an abdominal aortic aneurysm. Pain is not necessarily of sudden onset or extreme severity. Radiation to the back or flank and the association of an abdominal bruit should suggest this diagnosis.

Referred pain is usually from thorax, spine or genitalia, and may be accompanied by splinting of the hemidiaphragm, intensified by cough or sneezing and accentuated by local pressure, respectively. Myocardial infarction, pneumonia, pericarditis and oesophageal disease may present with abdominal pain and cause havoc with an unwary physician's reputation! Metabolic causes of abdominal pain, such as porphyria, are fortunately rare. Neurogenic causes have a burning character and are often in a peripheral nerve distribution. Hyperaesthesia is a common demonstrable feature.

Management of abdominal pain is exacting. An orderly, detailed history, paying great attention to the chronological sequence of events is essential. Careful, gentle, and thorough physical examination is required, including pelvic and rectal examination. Laboratory investigation should include haemoglobin, white cell count differential, mid-stream urine examination (MSU), chemistry including serum amylase, and liver function tests. Abdominal paracentesis is a safe and effective diagnostic procedure, especially following blunt trauma to the abdomen. Erect and supine abdominal x-rays are invaluable where the demonstration of free air, bowel dilatation, or gas in the biliary tree may be identified. Ultrasound is useful in visualizing localized collections of fluid, gallbladder and pancreas. Surgical or conservative treatment will depend on the diagnosis.

Abdominal paracentesis
(*also known as* Abdominocentesis) The surgical puncture of the abdominal cavity to aspirate fluid (abdominocentesis) for diagnostic purposes. Ascitic fluid is examined for protein, cell counts and culture. In certain circumstances, amylase, glucose, lactate dehydrogenase, cytology and culture for mycobacterium is indicated.

Abdominal tuberculosis
see *Tuberculosis of the gastrointestinal tract*

Abdominocentesis
see *Abdominal paracentesis*

Abdominoperineal resection
A radical operation devised for total resection of carcinoma of the rectum, leaving the patient with a permanent colostomy. See also *Rectal cancer*

Abdominoscopy
Examination of abdominal structures, particularly with a laparoscope, which is

an illuminated tubular instrument, passed through a small abdominal incision.

Abetalipoproteinaemia

(*also known as* Bassen-Kornzweig disease) An autosomal recessive disorder characterized by ataxia, steatorrhoea, atypical retinitis pigmentosa, acanthotic red cells and serum lipid abnormalities. In abetalipoproteinaemia the small bowel enterocytes contain multiple lipid droplets. Mild steatorrhoea is characteristic in the first two years of life. It is a rare condition found predominantly in Ashkenazi Jews. (Figure 2)

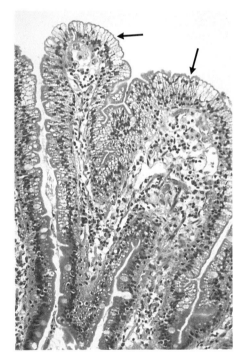

Figure 2 Abetalipoproteinaemia. Small intestinal villous epithelium showing vacuolation of enterocytes (arrowed) typical of abetalipoproteinaemia.

Abscess
A localized collection of pus in a cavity

formed by the disintegration of tissues associated with infection. Common bacteria involved include Gram-negative organisms (*Escherichia coli*, *Klebsiella proteus* and *Pseudomonas*), anaerobic bacteria (*Bacteroides*, *Clostridia* and anaerobic cocci) and amoebae (*Entamoeba histolytica*). Any part of the body can be affected with symptoms of localized swelling, redness, tenderness, generalized fever, and malaise. A leucocytosis is common, and septicaemia can occur. In gastroenterology, liver, appendix, sigmoid colon (with diverticulitis) and terminal ileum (with Crohn's disease) are the most common sites. Other sites include the anal region, biliary tract, pancreas and, rarely, caecum.

Table 1 Common types of abscess

Site	Clinical Features
Anorectal	Rectal pain, swelling and discharge
Appendiceal	Results from perforated appendix. Right iliac fossa mass, fever, malaise and tenderness
Biliary	Fever, jaundice and right upper quadrant pain radiating to the back
Epiploic (omental)	Epigastric mass
Hepatic	Right upper quadrant tenderness, fever, malaise
Mural	Abscess in abdominal wall. Redness, swelling and tenderness at site.
Pelvirectal	Lies above levator ani muscle. Symptoms as for Anorectal
Postcaecal	Lies posterior to caecum and may originate from appendix.
Subhepatic	Fever only. Can occur after surgery.

Absorption
The uptake of substances and fluids from the gastrointestinal tract at a cellular level, across the epithelial surface of the intestinal cell and hence into body tissues.

Absorption

The process of digestion is separate from absorption. Amino acids, mono- and disaccharides, monoglycerides and fatty acids are the end products of digestion and are absorbed in the small intestine where microscopic projections called villi greatly enhance the absorptive surface area.

Mechanisms There are four mechanisms considered important in intestinal absorption. *Active transport* is the transport of a substance across a cell membrane against a chemical or electrical gradient. It is energy dependent, carrier-mediated and subject to competitive inhibition. *Passive diffusion* occurs down an electrical or chemical gradient, is energy independent, and not subject to competitive inhibition. *Facilitated diffusion* is similar to passive diffusion, but is carrier-mediated and often subject to competitive inhibition. *Endocytosis* is similar to phagocytosis. Nutrients are enveloped by the outer plasma membrane of the cell. (Figure 3)

Sites of absorption Many substances are absorbed throughout the length of the small intestine. However, the proximal small intestine is the major area for absorption of iron, calcium, water soluble vitamins, and fat. Sugars are absorbed in both proximal and mid-small intestine while amino acids are preferentially absorbed in the mid-small intestine or jejunum. The ileum or distal small intestine absorbs most of the bile salts and vitamin B_{12}, while the colon is responsible for absorption of water and electrolytes. Abnormal absorption is present in a number of conditions affecting the small bowel, pancreas and liver. Malabsorption of food, nutrients and vitamins occurs. Symptoms include diarrhoea, steatorrhoea, weight loss, lethargy and malaise. A macrocytic anaemia, hypocalcaemia, iron deficiency and vitamin B_{12} deficiency may be seen on simple blood tests.

Biliary stage Bile acids solubilize fat by emulsification prior to action by pancreatic lipase and colipase and therefore assist absorption.
See also *Calcium absorption: Malabsorption*

Acalculous cholecystitis
see *Cholecystitis*

Acanthosis nigricans
A grey-black skin lesion, very suggestive of malignant disease, especially adeno-carcinoma of the stomach, when it develops in adults. Hyperpigmented raised, velvety lesions occur on the skin, and are associated with Cushing's syndrome and acromegaly as well as underlying malignancy.

Acetaminophen (paracetamol) poisoning
A common and potentially lethal condition which can lead to delayed hepatic damage and renal failure. Toxicity occurs with as little as 6-8 gms in a single dose, and is due to toxic metabolites of acetaminophen which deplete sulphydryl groups. N-acetylcysteine or cysteamine, within 10-12 hours of acetaminophen ingestion is effective therapy. Emesis or gastric lavage should be instituted immediately. Monitoring of the prothrombin time is the most sensitive indicator of prognosis. Raised transaminases are a common finding.

Table 2 Tests of absorption

Increased stool fat
Decreased serum albumin, calcium, iron, folate and vitamin B_{12}
Decreased xylose absorption
Abnormal lactose tolerance test
Anaemia, for example due to decreased iron, folate and vitamin B_{12}
Prolonged prothrombin time
Decreased vitamin B_{12} absorption
Abnormal pattern to barium follow-through
Abnormal small bowel biopsy

See also *individual tests*

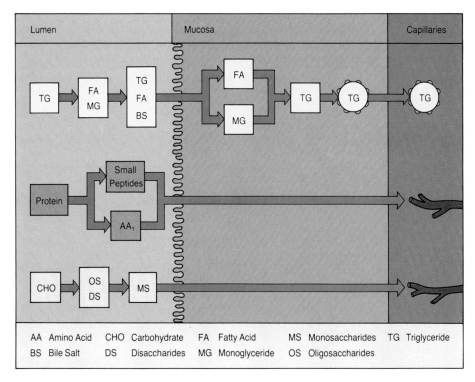

| AA | Amino Acid | CHO | Carbohydrate | FA | Fatty Acid | MS | Monosaccharides | TG | Triglyceride |
| BS | Bile Salt | DS | Disaccharides | MG | Monoglyceride | OS | Oligosaccharides | | |

Figure 3 **Absorption.** Diagram shows the absorption of protein, carbohydrates and fats via the enterocyte into capillaries and lymphatics.

Acetarsone (acetarsol)
A drug which contains arsenic used previously for amoebic dysentery, Vincent's angina, and spirochaetal infections. Skin rashes and irritation are recognized side-effects.

Achalasia
A motor disorder of the oesophagus, caused by failure of the relaxation mechanism of the lower oesophageal sphincter, and loss of normal peristalsis in the lower two-thirds of the oesophagus during swallowing. Symptoms include dysphagia, chest pain on swallowing, and regurgitation of food and fluid. Diagnosis is confirmed on barium swallow examination, and chest x-ray may reveal aspiration pneumonia. Pneumatic dilatation at endoscopy or surgical myotomy to disrupt the lower oesophageal sphincter is the appropriate treatment. Complications of long-standing achalasia include, pulmonary aspiration and carcinoma of the oesophagus. (Figure 4a and b)

Achalasia, pelvirectal
A rarely used term for congenital absence of ganglion cells in a distal segment of the large bowel. See also *Hirschsprung's disease.*

Achlorhydria
(*also known as* Gastric anacidity) An absence of hydrochloric acid from maximally stimulated gastric secretions. It is associated with both pernicious anaemia and chronic gastritis, as well as

gastric cancer and benign gastric ulcer disease. The presence of achlorhydria in a patient with a gastric ulcer increases the likelihood of gastric cancer.

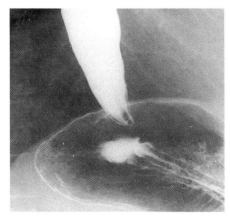

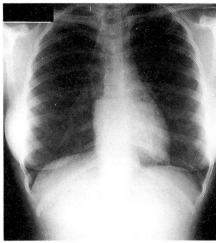

Figure 4a Achalasia. Barium swallow radiograph showing a moderately dilated oesophagus with smooth regular tapering at the gastro-oesophageal junction.
Figure 4b Achalasia. Erect chest x-ray showing a fluid level in the mid-oesophagus associated with proven achalasia.

Acholia
The deficiency or absence of the secretion of bile, which may be caused by an obstructed bile duct.

Acholuria (acholuric)
An absence of bile pigments in the urine, as in acholuric jaundice.

Achylia
An absence of secretion, commonly applied to the lack of hydrochloric acid and pepsinogens in the gastric juice.

Achymia
A lack of chyme.

Acidaemia
An abnormally high blood acidity which may occur in diabetic ketoacidosis, acute and chronic alcoholism and poisoning with salicylates, ethylene glycol and methyl alcohol. It may also result from acute loss of alkali, as in severe diarrhoea.

Acidosis
This is an excess acid or decreased alkaline reserve (bicarbonate content) in the blood and body tissues. This condition is characterized by an increase in hydrogen ion concentration (decrease in pH).

Acidosis (hyperchloraemic)
Metabolic acidosis is associated with elevated plasma chloride levels. It occurs in renal tubular acidosis where there is reduced excretion of acid and increased reabsorption of chloride to maintain electroneutrality.

Acinar units of the liver
Functional unit of the liver first envisaged by Rappaport. The unit is based on a portal triad with its terminal branch of portal vein, hepatic artery and bile duct. The circulatory limit of the acinus, near the central vein is most susceptible to injury, whether toxic, viral or anoxic, and this is where bridging necrosis occurs. (Figure 5)

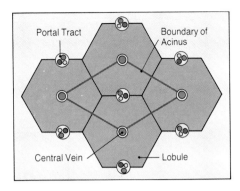

Figure 5 Acinar units of the liver. Diagram of the acinar unit of the liver as opposed to the lobular unit of the liver.

Acoprous
An intestine without faecal material.

Acquired immune deficiency syndrome
see *AIDS*

Acquired megacolon
see *Megacolon*

Acrodermatitis enteropathica
A rare disorder of dermatitis and diarrhoea due to zinc deficiency. Scaling and crusting skin lesions occur on the limbs, around the mouth and anus. The condition resolves quickly with oral or parenteral zinc replacement.

Actinomycosis, hepatic
An infection due to a fungus, *Actinomyces israelii*. It usually spreads to the liver from the caecum or appendix via the portal vein. Large localized collections of pus occur in the liver. The appropriate therapy is high dose penicillin for six weeks together with local instillation of penicillin, where possible.

Acute
A disease of sudden onset and severe symptoms, usually of brief duration. See also *Chronic: and specific disorders*

Acute yellow atrophy
(*also known as* Hepatodystrophy: Rokitansky's disease) An uncommon pathological finding in the liver after fulminant or viral hepatitis, or drug or carbon tetrachloride toxicity. There is extensive necrosis of the liver. Whereas the acute form is usually fatal, the subacute form involves less cellular damage, and has a better prognosis. However, subacute yellow atrophy of the liver may cause death from liver failure or progressive hepatic encephalopathy. See also *Cirrhosis: Hepatitis: Liver atrophy*

Adenoacanthoma
A mixed neoplasm exhibiting both glandular and squamous elements, the latter regarded as metaplastic. The term is generally restricted to benign lesions. It is rare and sites for the tumour include biliary tract, colon, duodenum, stomach, jejunum, anal region, oesophagus, pancreas and small intestine.

Adenocarcinoma
A malignant invasive neoplasm derived from the glandular epithelium constituting the gastrointestinal tract. The term can be further qualified by the degree of glandular differentiation, mucin production, and architectural features, such as a tubular, or papillary pattern. (Figure 6)

Adenoma
A mass of dysplastic glandular epithelium that is still benign. In hollow structures this will form a polyp and in solid organs a space occupying tumour.
Tubular adenoma More than 80% of the adenoma shows tubular formations
Villous adenoma More than 80% of the adenoma should demonstrate a finger-like growth pattern of the epithelium.
Tubular villous adenoma Mixture of the tubular and villous growth patterns such that each pattern exceeds 20%.
The most common site is in the large intestine but adenomas occur in the colon, gallbladder, stomach, islets of Langerhans,

Adenomatosis

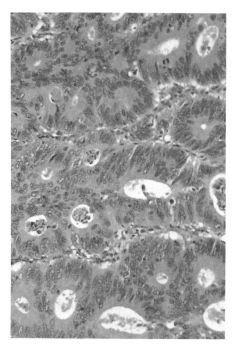

Figure 6 Adenocarcinoma. Microscopy showing crowded dysplastic glands of a typical well-differentiated adenocarcinoma (X25).

as well as in the liver and small intestine. (Figure 7a and b)

Adenomatosis
A condition characterized by development of numerous adenomas.

Adenomatosis (polyendocrine)
(*also known as* Multiple endocrine adenomatosis: Pluriglandular adenomatosis: Polyendocrinoma: Werner's syndrome) A rare syndrome involving adenomas or hyperplasia of more than one endocrine tissue; common sites include the anterior pituitary gland, the islets of Langerhans, and the parathyroid. See also *Zollinger-Ellison syndrome*

Adenomatous polyp
see *Polyp*

Adenomyoma of gallbladder
A benign localized area of adenomyosis which forms a recognizable tumour.

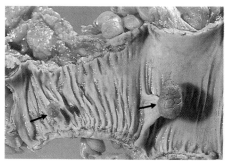

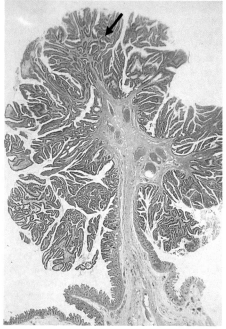

Figure 7a Adenoma. Colectomy showing two stalked adenomas (arrowed).
Figure 7b Adenoma. Histology showing dysplastic epithelium (arrowed) confined to the mucosa and not involving the stalk.

Adenomyomatosis of gallbladder
Diffuse outpouching of the lining epithelium of the gallbladder associated with proliferation of the surrounding muscle coat. See also *Rokitansky-Aschoff sinuses*

Adenosine arabinoside therapy
This is a drug used to combat DNA viruses and is given intramuscularly for four weeks. It is used in active hepatitis B infections which are e antigen positive. In this situation one third of patients convert their e antigen to anti-H Be but their HBsAg persists. Serum transaminases initially rise and then later fall in those patients who respond to treatment. Side-effects of treatment are muscular pains, headache, fever and malaise.

Adenosquamous carcinoma
A malignant neoplasm containing malignant glandular and malignant squamous epithelium.

Adenyl cyclase
An enzyme found in the liver and muscle cell membranes, which catalyzes the conversion of adenosine triphosphate (ATP) to cyclic adenosine monophosphate (AMP) plus pyrophosphate.

Adhesion
The union of two surfaces which are not normally applied together. Following abdominal surgery, fibrous bands may unite external bowel surfaces leading to colicky pain and possible obstruction of the bowel. Surgical division is the most appropriate treatment.

Adult hypertrophic pyloric stenosis
A rare condition of gastric outlet obstruction at the pylorus occurring in the adult. The anatomy and histology are indistinguishable from the infantile type. Clinical features include nausea, vomiting, epigastric pain, weight loss and anorexia. Careful investigation with barium meal and/or gastroscopy must distinguish it

from pyloric canal ulcer, antral cancer or duodenal ulcer. Treatment is surgical division or local resection. See also *Infantile hypertrophic pyloric stenosis: Pyloric stenosis*

Adult respiratory distress syndrome (ARDS), in acute pancreatitis
Many patients with severe acute pancreatitis have hypoxaemia. This may progress to severe hypoxia with tachypnoea, and diffuse pulmonary infiltrates, called adult respiratory distress syndrome, where hyaline membranes can be seen in the alveoli. It is associated with a poor prognosis. Patients may require corticosteroids and ventilatory assistance. See also *Pancreatitis*

Aerogastria
Gas present in the stomach, or a stomach bubble.

Aerophagia
(*also known as* Aerophagy: Gastrospiry)
The spasmodic swallowing of air followed by belching, which may be associated with functional gastrointestinal disturbance.

Aerophagy
see *Aerophagia*

Afferent loop syndrome
This is an acute syndrome which follows gastric surgery which has resulted in the construction of a blind loop. It occurs in the immediate postoperative period, is uncommon and presents with abdominal pain, vomiting and distension. It may resemble pancreatitis with raised serum amylase levels. Treatment is immediate surgical intervention. See also *Bacterial overgrowth*

Aflatoxin
A toxin from the mould *Aspergillus flavus*, which is associated with primary hepatic cancer in areas of Africa. Aflatoxin is ingested from contaminated food, such as groundnuts.

Agastria

Absence of the stomach.

Aglutition

Inability to swallow.

Agranulocytosis

(*also known as* Granulocytopenia: Schultz's disease) A disorder marked by a substantial decrease in the number of granulocytes (white cells) in the bone marrow and peripheral blood. It is accompanied by fever and ulceration of mucous membranes of the gastrointestinal tract and of the skin. It is associated with drugs, for example, chloramphenicol and carbimazole. Marrow recovery usually occurs if the patient can be maintained with barrier nursing, white cell transfusions, and general supportive treatment.

AIDS (acquired immune deficiency syndrome)

A syndrome, first reported in 1981, of lymphadenopathy, opportunistic infections, immunoparesis and Kaposi's syndrome, occurring in central Africa and Haiti, and now spreading throughout the Western world. Homosexual men are particularly at risk where blood-borne infection during anal intercourse is the likely mode of transmission. Other risk groups include female sexual partners of homosexual men, children born of infected mothers, intravenous drug abusers, and haemophiliacs using pooled blood products (factor VIII).

Cause The cause of this illness is the HIV infection (formerly HTLVIII/LAV virus). This virus is a retrovirus which causes immunosuppression, by infecting the T helper cells, a subset of peripheral blood lymphocytes. This acquired defect in cellular immunity leads to opportunistic infections, which may be viral, fungal or protozoal. Immunoparesis also leads to the development of certain tumours, notably Kaposi's sarcoma and non-Hodgkin's lymphoma.

Symptoms Infections with this virus may lead to a wide spectrum of illness, including persistent generalized lymphadenopathy, (PGL). Approximately 50% of these patients will ultimately develop AIDS. The majority, however, do not appear to have progressed in a 3-4 year follow up. Infection with HIV virus may lead to an acute generalized illness with fever, malaise, arthralgia, a maculo-papular rash and transient tender lymphadenopathy, lasting 2-3 weeks. The incubation period from exposure to onset of symptoms is probably 4-6 weeks, and seroconversion (IgG antibody) occurs at the time of generalized symptoms. The virus can be isolated from semen and saliva, although there is no evidence of transmission from saliva. Infection has been documented from a needle stick injury in a nurse. After infection, with or without symptoms, a period of latency follows when IgG antibodies remain positive and the virus can be isolated from peripheral blood lymphocytes. This period may last up to five years, but appears shorter in homosexual men or intravenous drug abusers. Persistent generalized lymphadenopathy (PGL) is a condition associated aetiologically with HIV virus infection. In New York, 25% of patients with PGL will develop frank AIDS over a 3-6 month period. A proportion of PGL patients will develop symptoms and signs of fever, sweats, weight loss and oral candidiasis, termed the AIDS related complex (ARC).

AIDS is manifested by the development of opportunistic infections, especially *Pneumocystis carinii* pneumonia and tumours. Over 70% of chest infections in AIDS are due to this organism, and a further 25% of patients present with Kaposi's sarcoma. Other important sites of infection occur in the gastrointestinal tract, the central nervous system and the skin. In the gastrointestinal tract, symptoms include persistent diarrhoea, abdominal colic, dysphagia and perianal discomfort. Signs of leukoplakia, *Candida* and Kaposi's sarcoma may be revealed in the mouth. Abdominal tenderness, splenomegaly, cachexia, and perianal ulceration may also be present. However, clinical signs may be absent or minimal, therefore a high index of suspicion is appropriate in at risk groups. There are several other infectious organisms associated with AIDS. Oral, oesophageal and gastric candidiasis is common in AIDS patients and the most effective treatment is ketoconazole. *Cryptosporidium* causes severe diarrhoea but unfortunately no specific treatment is available. The diagnosis is confirmed by staining the stool with an acid alcohol fast stain. Oral and perianal type 2 Herpes virus produces florid, painful and persistent ulcers. Cytomegalovirus may produce a colitis by invading the colonic mucosa. Finally, AIDS patients are also susceptible to *Salmonella*.

Prevention HIV has low infectivity and is far less infectious than hepatitis B. However, because of its devastating effects, guidelines to prevent its spread from patient to patient, and patient to health worker, have been produced. Disinfection of endoscopes, screening of blood donors, advice to nurses and laboratory staff, and appropriate education for at risk groups, are essential to meeting and defeating this unique disease.

Alactasia
Absence or reduction of the small bowel brush border enzyme lactase. It may occur following bouts of severe diarrhoea and in childhood *de novo*. Symptoms include cramp, abdominal pain, milk intolerance and diarrhoea. Diagnosis is confirmed with a lactose tolerance test, and treatment is a lactose-free diet.

Alanine transaminase (ALT)
An enzyme within the cytoplasm of liver cells which increases with liver cell damage, as in hepatitis. A rise in the level is a more specific indicator of liver damage than aspartate transaminase (AST), but the absolute rise is quantitatively less than AST.

Albumin
A water-soluble protein synthesized by the liver and forming a major protein fraction in the blood. The main function of albumin is to maintain plasma volume by colloid oncotic pressure, but it also binds and transports many substances, including hormones, fatty acids, trace metals, bilirubin and calcium. It is produced by the liver at approximately 12gm/day (the half-life of serum albumin is 17-20 days) and a normal serum level is 3.5-5.0 gm/dl. Low levels of albumin are associated with cirrhosis of the liver, malabsorption and nephrotic syndrome. In refractory ascites, infusion of salt poor albumin may initiate a temporary diuresis.

Albuminocholia
Albumin present in the bile.

Albuminorrhoea
Excessive faecal excretion of albumin.

Alcohol and liver disease
The chronic ingestion of large quantities of alcohol (ethyl alcohol) leads to liver damage in susceptible individuals. This may take the form of fatty infiltration (alcoholic steatosis), alcoholic hepatitis, or cirrhosis. Histological progression from steatosis to cirrhosis is reduced, but not abolished, by abstinence. Women are more susceptible to developing cirrhosis with the same amount of alcohol than men, and the severity of the initial liver lesion influences the development of cirrhosis.

Pathogenesis Ethanol is oxidized, mainly in the liver, to acetaldehyde, which is likely to contribute to tissue damage associated with the abuse of alcohol. Acetaldehyde is a very active compound capable of binding to plasma proteins, microsomal proteins, the free amino acids and sulphydryl groups of haemoglobin. Metabolism of acetaldehyde produces nicotinamide adenine dinucleotide

Alcohol malabsorption

(NADH) which may contribute to tissue damage associated with excess alcohol ingestion. Enhanced lipid oxidation may be a mechanism for alcohol induced fatty liver, and this is accentuated in animals by selenium deficiency. Abnormal fibrogenesis and the direct effect of alcohol on membrane lipid may also be important in pathogenesis.

Diagnosis is dependent on a careful history and examination, (findings showing signs of chronic liver disease, such as jaundice, palmar erythema, pale nails, spider naevae, hepatomegaly or ascites), and abnormal liver function tests with raised aspartate transaminase and gamma glutamyl transpeptidase. The liver biopsy is the cornerstone of accurate diagnosis, and is of prognostic significance.

Treatment Nitrogen balance has been shown in clinical trials to be an important aspect of treatment, because many of these patients are malnourished. The development of alcoholic hepatitis carries a high mortality and may be related to binge drinking. Abstinence from alcohol is a constant battle for the patient, and regular, careful follow-up, with repeat liver function tests and periodic blood or urine alcohol estimations are useful clinical indicators of relapse. Open discussion, and sensitive consistent encouragement is important to get these patients back to a useful productive lifestyle. See also *Fetal alcohol syndrome*

Alcohol malabsorption
In moderate amounts, alcohol produces direct structural damage to cells of the upper small intestine, with impairment of absorption of amino acids and thiamine. Chronic ingestion impairs sodium and water transport. Steatorrhoea seen in alcoholics is related to exocrine pancreatic disease. See also *Malabsorption*

Alcoholic myopathy
Type II muscle fibre atrophy is associated with alcoholism. Wasting mainly affects proximal muscle groups.

Aldosterone
Raised levels of aldosterone increase sodium absorption and potassium excretion from the colon similar to the effect of aldosterone on the kidney.

Alginate
The salt of alginic acid, when soluble, forms a viscous layer on top of the stomach contents preventing acid reflux into the lower oesophagus. It is useful in treatment of oesophagitis with reflux of acid or bile. See also *Oesophagitis*

Alimentary canal
(*also known as* Gastrointestinal tract) Canal from the mouth to the anus along which food passes allowing digestion, nutrient absorption and finally, excretion of waste products. (Figure 8)

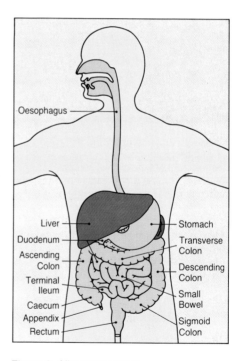

Figure 8 Alimentary canal.

Alimentation, parenteral
see *Parenteral alimentation (nutrition)*

Alkali
A substance that can accept hydrogen ions or proteins in aqueous solution. It turns red litmus blue and is corrosive to tissue.

Alkali injury to upper gastrointestinal tract
Ingested alkali can cause progressive and severe injury to the stomach and the oesophagus. Since alkali cleansers were introduced in the 1960s, this problem has increased. Oesophageal strictures and gastric stenosis can occur. Alkali may cause full thickness necrosis and inflammation of the oesophagus and stomach. Acute symptoms include persistent salivation, dysphagia, or even hoarseness and stridor, dyspnoea and shock. Gastric and oesophageal perforation can occur with signs of mediastinitis or peritonitis. Management includes preventing vomiting, fasting, and general supportive measures. Neutralization with acids causes an exothermic reaction which may increase tissue damage.

Alkaline phosphatase
An enzyme present in a number of tissues including liver, bile canaliculi, bone, intestine and placenta. Serum levels mainly reflect a bony or hepatic origin. A distinction between these two sources can be made by fractionation or measurement of gamma glutamyl transpeptidase and 5-nucleotidase. These are concomitantly raised alongside the alkaline phosphatase in liver disease.

Alkaline reflux
see *Gastritis*

Alkalosis (metabolic)
see *Metabolic alkalosis*

Allergic proctitis
Lubricants used during anal intercourse can irritate the rectal mucosa and cause contact sensitivity. The term has also been applied to a limited proctitis with increased numbers of IgE containing plasma cells.

Allergy, and intestinal disease
A disorder where the body becomes hypersensitive to certain antigens. There are three main patterns of allergic disorders of the intestine:
Eosinophilic gastroenteritis is a disorder of the stomach and/or small bowel, associated with eosinophilic infiltration of the gut wall and eosinophilia in the blood. Patients may show specific food intolerance, malabsorption and gastrointestinal symptoms on blind food challenge. Elimination of specific food, or treatment with steroids improves symptoms and histological changes.
Food allergy in childhood. Milk intolerance with vomiting and diarrhoea is the most common form.
Food intolerance with anaphylactic reactions are, fortunately, very rare. See also *Eosinophilic gastroenteritis: Food allergy: Food intolerance*. (Table 3)

Allochezia
The excretion of nonfaecal matter.

Alpha-1-antitrypsin
An acute phase plasma protein (an alpha-1-globulin) produced in the liver, inhibiting the activity of trypsin and other proteolytic enzymes.

Alpha-1-antitrypsin deficiency (α-1-AT)
Alpha-1-antitrypsin is an ubiquitous acute-phase protein which protects tissues from enzymatic degradation. Deficiency of this protein is caused by an inherited autosomal dominant condition with disease affecting both lung (emphysema) and liver (neonatal hepatitis and progressive cirrhosis). Fortunately, only 10% of infants with homozygous genetics will have liver involvement. No specific

Table 3 Classification and clinical patterns of allergic diseases of the intestine and eosinophilic gastroenteritis

A Eosinophilic gastroenteritis criteria for diagnosis
Infiltration of gut wall with eosinophils
Increased number of eosinophils in peripheral blood

B Clinical patterns of allergic diseases
Predominant mucosal disease
Predominant muscle layer disease
Predominant subserosal disease
Combinations of the above

C Allergic gastroenteritis in childhood
Milk intolerance in infancy and childhood
Soy protein allergy
Gluten enteropathy

D Gastrointestinal food intolerance with systemic allergic reactions

treatment is available. Heterozygotes have 10% of normal serum α-1-AT level, and can remain well throughout life or may develop emphysema. Hepatocytes in a liver biopsy show characteristic globules staining red by periodic acid Schiff (PAS) method.

Alpha-1-fetoprotein (AFP)
A protein normally found in the plasma of human fetuses from six weeks to birth. Elevated levels occur in primary liver cancer and this is a useful marker of this condition. It is also present in the serum of patients with ovarian and testicular malignancies. Ninety per cent of primary liver cancer patients are positive using a radioimmunoassay method for detection. See also *Liver cancer*

Alpha heavy chain disease, and intestinal lymphoma
A disease characterized by malabsorption and plasma cell infiltration of the small bowel wall which can progress to a malignant lymphoma. Incomplete IgA heavy chains are seen in the serum and urine of patients. Presenting symptoms include abdominal pain, weight loss and malabsorption. In a few patients antibiotics have improved symptoms. The disease is usually found in patients between the ages of 10 and 30.

Alprostadil
A vasodilator. See also *Prostaglandins*

Aluminium hydroxide
A white, amorphous powder, used as an antacid to treat peptic ulcer and dyspepsia, in the form of aluminium hydroxide gel or dried aluminium hydroxide gel. It reacts in the stomach to form aluminium chloride. It may cause reduced absorption of iron and tetracyclines and can lead to constipation. See also *Antacids*

American trypanosomiasis
see *Chagas' disease*

Amiloride
A potassium-sparing diuretic useful in the treatment of ascites. See also *Diuretics in ascites*

Amine precursor uptake and decarboxylation cells
see *APUD cells*

Amino acids, in liver disease
Organic compounds containing an amino (NH_2) and a carboxyl group (COOH). Aromatic amino acids are increased in liver disease probably due to reduced hepatic deamination.

Ammonia toxicity and hepatic encephalopathy

Ammonia is metabolized by the liver to urea. In hepatic encephalopathy, blood ammonia levels rise and ammonium can cross the blood-brain barrier, causing depression of the cerebral blood flow and glucose metabolism. Blood ammonia levels usually correlate with severity of coma.

Amoeba

A single-celled nucleated protozoon of the subphylum Sarcodina.

Amoebiasis

An infectious disease prevalent in the tropics due to amoebic infection, especially *Entamoeba histolytica*, which leads to both an acute and chronic disease with multiple organs involved, especially the colon, liver and lungs. Clinically the spectrum of disease is wide, varying from asymptomatic to a severe prostrating illness with mucosal ulceration and perforation.

In the human colon, *Entamoeba histolytica* exists in the trophozoite form (motile) and in cysts (non-motile). Cysts are the infective agent and are excreted in the stool. On ingestion, the cyst forms trophozoites and lodges in the colon leading to amoebic colitis.

Clinical symptoms include abdominal pain, intermittent diarrhoea, anorexia and malaise.

Diagnosis is by repeated microscopic examination of 3-6 fresh stools.

Treatment with metronidazole (750 mg three times daily for 7-10 days) followed by diiodohydroxyquinoline (650 mg three times daily for 20 days) is usually adequate. (Figure 9) See also *Amoebic colitis: Amoebicides*

Amoebic colitis

Inflammation of the colon due to *Entamoeba histolytica*, in which there is colonic ulceration presenting with rectal bleeding, abdominal pain and fever. It must

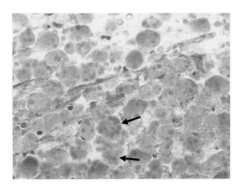

Figure 9 Amoebiasis. A large number of amoebic trophozoites are seen, many with ingested red blood corpuscles (arrowed).

be distinguished from ulcerative colitis and Crohn's disease by rectal biopsy, and assessment of stool for cysts. Serum should be sent for an amoebic complement fixation test. See also *Amoebiasis: Colitis*

Amoebic dysentery

see *Dysentery*

Amoebic liver abscess

The liver is the most common extra-intestinal site for this abscess and if untreated it is often fatal. Metronidazole and diiodohydroxyquinoline in combination is very effective. Needle aspiration may be useful for large abscesses but surgical drainage is usually not indicated. Chest involvement may occur either with direct spread from the liver through the diaphragm or secondary to intestinal involvement. See also *Abscess*

Amoebicides

Agents which are destructive to amoebae. *Metronidazole* is active against *Entamoeba histolytica* as trophozoites, cysts and liver abscess. However, it is not as effective against organisms within the bowel lumen. It should be used in all types of amoebiasis either alone or in combination with other drugs.

Amoeboma

Diiodohydroxyquinoline acts against intraluminal amoebae. It is suitable treatment in conjunction with metronidazole for intestinal amoebiasis. *Diloxanide furoate* is active against cysts and is a safe treatment for asymptomatic cyst carriers.

Other amoebicides include: Metronidazole analogues, for example emetine hydrochloride, iodoquinol, ornidazole and tinidazole, dehydroemetine, paromomycin sulphate and tetracycline.

Amoeboma

A tumour-like mass produced by localized inflammation due to amoebiasis.

Ampulla of Vater

(Abraham Vater, German anatomist 1684-1751)
The dilatation formed by junction of the common bile and the pancreatic duct proximal to their opening into the duodenum.

Amylase

An enzyme that occurs in saliva and pancreatic secretions to aid digestion of starch. Serum levels are raised in acute pancreatitis and in parotitis. Amylase is an excellent screening test for acute pancreatitis.

Amylase creatinine clearance ratio, in acute pancreatitis

During the course of acute pancreatitis, there is early excretion of amylase compared with creatinine. The amylase creatinine ratio (ACR) =

$$\frac{\text{Amylase urine} \times \text{Creatinine serum}}{\text{Amylase serum} \times \text{Creatinine urine}} \times \frac{100}{1}$$

Normal range is 1-4%. In acute pancreatitis levels of more than 4% occur. It is non-specific and offers no advantage over a serum amylase level.

Amyloid

An extracellular fibrillar protein formed by proteolysis of a protein precursor, yielding a characteristic twisted beta-pleated sheet structure. It is recognized grossly by its waxy hyaline appearance and microscopically by its eosinophilia, metachromatic staining, and dichroism. It is stained red with Congo red and then gives a diagnostic green birefringence under polarized light. It has a diagnostic fibrillar pattern on electron microscopy.

Amyloid disease

(*also known as* Amyloidosis) A syndrome due to deposition of the extracellular fibrillar protein amyloid. It may be primary, when no underlying cause is found, or secondary to another disease, for example, multiple myeloma, chronic infections such as tuberculosis or osteomyelitis, rheumatoid arthritis, or familial Mediterranean fever. Clinically, multiple sites can be involved, including gastrointestinal tract, liver, kidney, heart, skin, nervous system, joints and respiratory systems. The gastrointestinal involvement may present with malabsorption, abdominal pain, intestinal obstruction, or protein-losing enteropathy. Deposition of amyloid is seen primarily in vessel walls and any part of the gastrointestinal tract may be affected but deep rectal biopsy is a relatively reliable, safe means of diagnosis. Up to 80% of patients may be diagnosed by this method with submucosal vessel being sampled. Macroglossia occurs in 15-20% of patients due to amyloid infiltration of the tongue. Colonic involvement may present with diarrhoea, constipation, megacolon or faecal incontinence. Therapy is unfortunately unrewarding. (Figure 10a and b)

Amyloidosis

see *Amyloid disease*

Amylorrhoea

The presence of starch in the stools.

Anaemia

A reduction of circulating red blood cells below normal values (12 gm/dl). Causes include decreased red cell production, increased red cell destruction and blood loss, which may be acute or chronic. Long-standing chronic diseases, such as rheumatoid arthritis, may be associated with anaemia. In Crohn's disease and ulcerative colitis, anaemia is related to disease activity. In peptic ulcer, anaemia is secondary to blood loss, while in pernicious anaemia, loss of intrinsic factor from the stomach results in loss of vitamin B_{12} absorption at the terminal ileum. In coeliac disease, anaemia is due to reduced absorption of iron or folate from the small intestine. Symptoms of anaemia include weakness, dyspnoea and palpitations following exercise and may progress to vertigo, headache and syncope. Anaemia is not a diagnosis, but its cause requires appropriate investigation. See also *Haemolytic anaemia*

Anaerobic organisms

These are organisms which grow in the absence of oxygen. Such organisms can be pathogenic, causing liver abscesses, gastroenteritis, and septicaemia. They can be difficult to grow in the laboratory as many are fastidious and require special media for their culture. Examples include, bacteroides species, *Clostridium tetani*, aerobacteria, and some streptococcal species.

Anal canal

This is the terminal 2½-3 cm of the alimentary canal. It is separated from

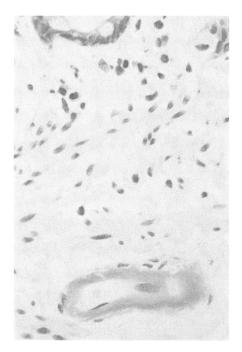

Figure 10a Amyloid disease. Rectal mucosa with amyloid in a submucosal vessel. This stains red with Congo red.

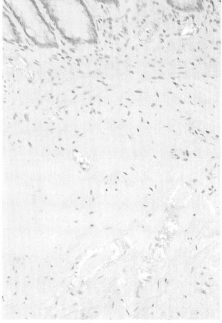

Figure 10b Amyloid disease. Rectal mucosa with amyloid exhibiting green birefringence when viewed in polarized light.

Anal fissure

the rectum by longitudinal mucosal folds at the dentate line and ends at the mucocutaneous junction (the pectinate line). The canal is surrounded by muscular sphincters and an extension of the levator ani which preserve continence. (Figure 11) See also *Anus*

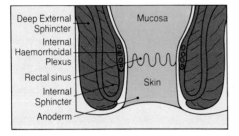

Figure 11 Anal canal.

Anal fissure

A longitudinal defect in the anal mucosa, mostly occurring in the midline posteriorly and usually due to the passage of large firm stools. Local pain on defaecation is severe and may be associated with bright red rectal bleeding. Treatment is by local soothing suppositories, softening of the stool, or surgical intervention (excision or dilatation).

Anal fistula

(*also known as* Anorectal fistula: Fistula in ano) This is a tract lined with granulation tissue connecting the anus or rectum with the perianal skin. The patient presents with drainage of pus, blood or mucus, and underlying causes such as Crohn's disease should be sought. Surgical treatment is required.

Anal skin tags

These are very common and consist of excess anal or perianal tissue. Occasionally they are a marker of an underlying anal disease, such as haemorrhoids or Crohn's disease.

Anal sphincter

The internal anal sphincter consists of circular smooth muscle. The external anal sphincter is a sheet of striated muscle, which lies in two positions both deep and superficial to the internal sphincter. The function of the anal sphincter is to preserve continence together with the levator ani muscles.

Analgesic(s) for diverticulosis

Antispasmodic drugs, for example hyoscine butylbromide are usually sufficient to relieve pain in diverticular disease. However, occasionally analgesics will be required and pethidine is the drug of choice. Pentazocine reduces sigmoid motility in analgesic doses, but side-effects of confusion, disorientation, and sometimes, hallucinations, especially in the elderly, make it less acceptable. See also *Diverticulosis*

Anastomosis

An artificial connection between two hollow organs which applies in gastro-enterology to two normally separate parts of intestine. These are defined by their locations, such as, ileorectal, Roux-en-Y, rectosigmoid and jejunocolic anastomoses. See also *individual anastomoses*

Ancylostomiasis

see *Hookworm disease*

Androgenic hormones

These virilizing compounds, especially C17 substituted testosterone, can cause hepatic adenoma and hepatocellular carcinoma. Up to 30% of patients treated with methyl testosterone may show abnormal liver function tests.

Aneurysm

An abnormal swelling of the wall of an artery which may be caused by atherosclerosis, idiopathic degeneration of the vessel wall, trauma, vasculitis, especially polyarteritis nodosa, infection

(mycotic aneurysm), or syphilis.
There are two main situations where aneurysms are relevant in gastroenterology:

Abdominal aortic aneurysm Most commonly of atherosclerotic origin, this aneurysm occurs below the level of the renal arteries and is found incidentally on physical examination, as a pulsatile mass accompanied by a bruit. Occasionally, symptoms of abdominal pain, back pain, or claudication, may be present. Diagnosis is confirmed by plain abdominal x-ray, ultrasound, or CT scan of the aorta. Prognosis depends on size, which if above 5 cm should be considered for surgical removal with replacement by a synthetic graft. Rupture occurs in about 10% of patients. (Figure 12)

Hepatic artery aneurysm This is rare and may occur after liver biopsy or cholecystectomy. It presents with right upper quadrant pain and fever and, if the common bile duct is affected, jaundice. Angiographic embolization is the treatment of choice.

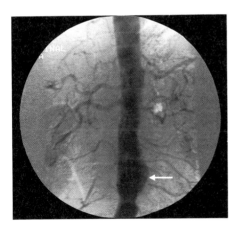

Figure 12 Aneurysm. Digital subtraction angiogram showing the abdominal aorta with an irregular aneurysmal dilatation (arrowed).

Aneurysmectomy

Surgical treatment for symptomatic or large aneurysms, usually of the abdominal aorta.

Angina (abdominal)

see *Abdominal (intestinal) angina*

Angiodysplasia

(*also known as* Arteriovenous malformation: Vascular dysplasia or ectasia) This is a localized arteriovenous malformation occurring mainly in the caecum or ascending colon. The histology shows foci of ectatic veins in the submucosa of the colon, with or without ectasia of overlying mucosal capillaries. Clinically the patient presents with painless lower gastrointestinal tract bleeding which can be massive but more commonly is slow and chronic with a history of previous episodes of bleeding or anaemia. The age range is 40-80 years and diagnosis is by colonoscopy and selective mesenteric angiography. Right hemicolectomy is the treatment of choice. However, between 5% and 37% of patients continue to bleed after surgery. (Figure 13a and b)

Angiography

A specialized radiological examination of arteries in which radio-opaque contrast is injected and several rapid films are taken outlining the vessels. Angiography is useful in the diagnosis and, more recently, treatment of acute gastro-intestinal bleeding. It is usually preceded by endoscopy and a trial of medical supportive therapy. A positive result will only be obtained if there is active bleeding at the time of the angiogram.
Therapeutic angiography involves both intra-arterial infusion of vasoconstrictor substances, such as vasopressin, and the newer vaso-occlusive therapy with Gelfoam. Angiography is also useful in the diagnosis, localization, and determination of operability in hepatocellular carcinoma.

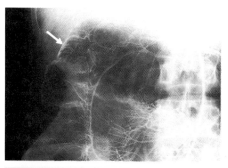

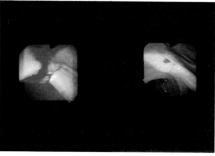

Figure 13a Angiodysplasia. Selective angiograph in the arterial phase showing angiodysplasia at the hepatic flexure. Note the network of small arterioles at the anti-mesenteric border of the hepatic flexure (arrowed).
Figure 13b Angiodysplasia. Actively bleeding duodenal angiodysplasia (left). The same lesion six weeks after successful diathermy (right).

Annular pancreas
A congenital abnormality of the pancreas where the ventral pancreas may encircle the duodenum leading to obstruction. The annulus is proximal to the ampulla of Vater, and usually involves the second part of the duodenum. Surgical treatment with duodenostomy or duodenojejunostomy is sometimes required. (Figure 14)

Anoperineal fistula
A congenital malformation between anus and perineum, localized, in the male, anywhere between the perineoscrotal

junction and the anal dimple. In the female any part of the vagina may be involved.

Anorectal fistula
see *Anal fistula*

Anorectal gonorrhoea
see *Gonorrhoea*

Anorectal manometry
Small balloons are inserted into the rectum and anus and the pressure is recorded. The internal sphincter pressure (3-7 cm from the anal verge) measures 25-85 cm of water. At defaecation, the pressure decreases and following it there is some rebound increase in pressure, called the closing reflex.

Anorexia
Loss of the appetite and lack of any desire to eat. It can occur with organic or psychological disorders and may be associated with other gastrointestinal symptoms such as vomiting, weight loss, abdominal pain, diarrhoea, or melaena. Anorexia is associated with other medical disorders, for example thyroid disease, congestive cardiac failure, chronic renal failure, and acute hepatitis, and is a side-effect of many drugs, such as

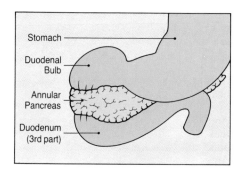

Figure 14 Annular pancreas. Diagramatic representation of an annular pancreas showing constriction of the second part of the duodenum by the head of the annular pancreas.

salazopyrin, or a symptom of toxicity, such as digoxin.

Anorexia nervosa

A disease mainly of girls and young women, with anorexia, profound weight loss, and amenorrhoea. The symptoms relate to severe psychological disturbance about food intake, and abnormal patterns of eating, such as food cramming followed by bulimia, are common. Initial motivation for weight loss is often obesity just prior to puberty. Hyperactivity is the rule. There is a spectrum of severity and in the severest form both gastroenterologist and psychiatrist should manage these patients jointly. Family therapy and restoring proper nutrition are useful early objectives. The mortality from starvation can be as high as 6%.

Anoscope

see *Proctoscope*

Anoscopy

see *Proctoscopy*

Anosigmoidoscopy

see *Proctosigmoidoscopy*

Antacid

A substance that neutralizes acidity, usually of the stomach. Antacids react with gastric acid to form salts and water. They are useful in the treatment of dyspepsia and peptic ulcer and in high dosage (30 ml 1 hr and 3 hrs after meals and 60 ml at night) have been shown by endoscopy to heal peptic ulcers. In this dosage they keep gastric pH greater than 2.0. Antacids relieve symptoms of dyspepsia and pain quickly and effectively. Only small amounts are absorbed by the gut. Antacids can cause side-effects. For instance, magnesium hydroxide can cause diarrhoea, while aluminium hydroxide sometimes leads to constipation. Large amounts of calcium carbonate can cause hypercalcaemia, and aluminium hydroxide must be used cautiously in renal failure where significant absorption may lead to aluminium toxicity.

Antiamoebics

Drugs that kill or suppress the growth of amoebae. Metronidazole and its derivatives are effective against trophozoites in stool cysts, and in extraintestinal sites. However, it may not be totally effective against organisms in the lumen of the bowel. Diiodochlorhydroxyquinoline is effective against intraluminal amoebae and it therefore is often used with metronidazole.

Antibiotics

Drugs which are either bactericidal, where the drug (for example, penicillin) alone is capable of destroying the organism, or bacteriostatic, where the drug (for example, sulphonamides) inhibits growth allowing the immune system to eradicate the organism. Antibiotics are required in many gastrointestinal complaints such as cholangitis, where ampicillin or mezlocillin in combination with an aminoglycoside drug, such as gentamicin is useful. Non-absorbable antibiotics, for example, neomycin, are useful in hepatic encephalopathy. Vancomycin or metronidazole are the drugs of choice in pseudomembranous colitis, while erythromycin is effective against campylobacter gastroenteritis.

Anticholelithogenic agents

Agents that prevent the formation of gallstones, such as chenodeoxycholic acid and ursodeoxycholic acid. They are used when surgery is inadvisable, symptoms are mild, gallstones are small (less than 1 cm) and radiolucent, and gallbladder function is normal. Successful dissolution of gallstones takes 6 months to 4 years, with one trial showing only a 14% success rate. Side-effects include diarrhoea and hepatotoxicity.

Anticholinergic drugs
These drugs block the muscarinic action of acetylcholine on structures supplied by cholinergic nerve endings. Conventional anticholinergic drugs are of little practical importance as dosage is limited by atropine-like side-effects. Pirenzepine is a new selective anticholinergic drug which reduces gastric secretion, and is effective in healing peptic ulcers. Anticholinergic drugs (for example, atropine) inhibit pepsin secretion but have complex multiple effects on serum gastrin and gastric emptying depending on dosage.

Antidiarrhoeal agents
Agents that are effective in controlling diarrhoea. They include codeine phosphate and loperamide, which reduce frequency and volume of stool, probably by reducing intestinal motility and thus facilitating absorption. Caution must be taken in patients with inflammatory bowel disease as antidiarrhoeal agents can precipitate toxic megacolon. See also *Codeine phosphate: Loperamide*

Antiemetic agents
These agents prevent nausea and vomiting, for example, metoclopramide improves gastric emptying, while prochlorperazine acts on the vomiting centre to depress activity. Antihistamines are useful for motion sickness.

Antigens
These are substances recognized by the body as foreign and against which antibodies are produced. Antigens are usually proteins. In hepatitis B a specific virus (hepatitis B virus) is the cause and the whole virus as well as viral particles are antigenic. See also *Hepatitis B antigens*

Antihistamine
(*also known as* Antihistaminic) Drug counteracting the action of histamine. There are two histamine receptors, H_1 *receptors* are blocked by conventional antihistamine drugs used for treatment of allergies, H_2 *receptor antagonists* are used in the treatment of peptic ulceration, because they cause a reduction in gastric acid secretion. See also H_2 *antagonists*: *Histamine*

Antilithic agents
Agents that prevent the formation of a calculus. See also *Anticholelithogenic agents*

Antimesenteric
The part of the intestine which is opposite the site of attachment of the mesentery.

Antimitochondrial antibody
Circulating serum antibodies against mitochondria are found in virtually all patients with primary biliary cirrhosis. It is unlikely that they are involved in pathogenesis. They may also occur in patients with chronic active hepatitis. See also *Cirrhosis*

Antinuclear factor in chronic active lupoid hepatitis
A non-specific autoantibody present in the serum of 80% of patients with chronic active lupoid hepatitis, and which correlates with gamma globulin levels in the serum. The antibody is also present in systemic lupus erythematosus.

Antiperistalsis
Reversed peristalsis. See also *Peristalsis*

Antireflux operations
The need for these operations has greatly diminished with the advent of H_2 receptor antagonists. The operation is designed to prevent the reflux of gastric contents into the oesophagus. There are many different techniques, but the main aim is to increase lower oesophageal sphincter tone by either invaginating the oesophagus into the stomach, or wrapping the fundus of the stomach around the oesophagus. Surgical therapy is usually applied only

for the complications of reflux (stricture formation, significant bleeding and pulmonary aspiration). Operations for hiatus herniae correction have left cases of reflux unaffected. Recent techniques aim to enhance closure of the gastro-oesophageal junction by invaginating the oesophagus into itself (Belsey operation) or by creation of a gastric wrap-around (Hills and Nissen procedures). There is considerable difference of opinion as to which procedure is the better although evidence to date tends to support the Nissen procedure.

Antisecretory drugs
These drugs antagonize gastric acid secretion and are used for the treatment of peptic ulceration. They fall into three main categories:
H₂ receptor antagonists inhibit basal and nocturnal acid secretion, as well as secretion stimulated by pentagastrin, histamine, insulin, hypoglycaemia, caffeine and food. It is thought that they inhibit the effect of histamine on parietal cell receptors. See also *H₂ antagonists*
Anticholinergic drugs antagonize the action of acetylcholine on cholinergic nerve fibres. See also *Anticholinergic drugs*
Prostaglandins and *tricyclic anti-depressants* suppress gastric acid secretion. These are drugs which reduce gastric acid secretion and are used for the treatment of peptic ulcer. Omeprazole, a benzimidazole, is a new (and as yet experimental) antisecretory agent acting directly on the ATPase of the gastric mucosa. It is a very potent inhibitor of gastric acid secretion, and may prove useful in Zollinger-Ellison syndrome. See also *Prostaglandins*: *Tricyclic antidepressants*

Antispasmodic agents
These drugs relieve tonic contraction of smooth muscle of the gut, bile duct, arteries or bronchi. In gastroenterology, antispasmodic drugs (for example,

hyoscine butylbromide and mebeverine hydrochloride), are useful in the treatment of acute biliary colic, diverticular disease, and irritable bowel disease. In radiological investigation of the gastrointestinal tract, hyoscine butylbromide is often used to relax the pyloric antral region and colon in order to reduce motility and therefore improve the radiograph quality. Side-effects of antispasmodic drugs include drowsiness, dry mouth, and blurring of vision.

Antitrypsin, α-1
see *Alpha-1-antitrypsin*

Antrectomy
This procedure involves the resection of the pyloric antrum of the stomach for surgical treatment of benign or malignant antral gastric ulcer.

Antroduodenectomy
This procedure involves the surgical removal of the pyloric antrum and adjacent part of the duodenum, previously used in the treatment of duodenal ulcer.

Antrum, gastric
The distal part of stomach extending from the incisura to the pylorus. See also *Stomach*

Anus
The orifice at the end of the alimentary canal. See also *Anal canal*

Aortic graft-duodenal fistula (aortoduodenal fistula)
A fistula between the proximal anastomosis of an aortic graft and usually the 3rd or 4th part of the duodenum. A herald bleed is common and concomitant back pain is a clue to the diagnosis. Urgent endoscopy is indicated and occasionally will reveal the site of bleeding. More importantly, other causes of bleeding should be assessed and if none found then it is assumed that the fistula is present and operation performed. Arteriography does

not usually show the fistula unless a false aneurysm, or active bleeding, is present.

Aorto-enteric fistula
see *Arterial-enteric fistula*

Aperistalsis
A lack of peristalsis.

Aphagia
Abstention from eating or inability to swallow.

Aphtha
see *Aphthous ulcers*

Aphthous ulcers
(*also known as* Aphtha) Small ulcers occurring in the mouth. Similar lesions seen elsewhere in the gastrointestinal tract as white or red spots are termed *aphthoid ulcers*. The cause is not known, but in coeliac disease and Crohn's disease there is a higher incidence. (Figure 15)

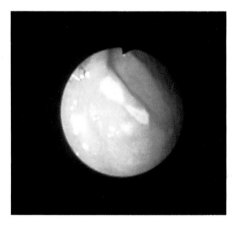

Figure 15 Aphthous ulcer. Colonoscopic view of two aphthoid ulcers in Crohn's disease seen as flat white ulcerated lesions.

Apnoea, deglutition
Temporary cessation of breathing due to arrest of the activity of the respiratory nerve centre during swallowing.

Appendectomy (appendicectomy)
Surgical removal of the appendix, usually for acute appendicitis. See also *Appendicitis*

Appendicitis (acute)
The peak incidence of acute appendicitis occurs between the ages of 10-30 years and affects males and females equally. Perforation, with either localized abscess formation or peritonitis, is much more common in infancy and in the elderly, where the diagnosis is more easily overlooked with a consequent increase in mortality. Appendicitis is extremely common, occurring in 7-12% of people during their lifetime.

Pathogenesis Appendicitis may be due to obstruction of the vermiform appendix, but this is observed in only 30-40% of cases. It is now thought that ulceration of the mucosa is the initial event in the majority of patients. Infection with bacteria and invasion of the wall of the appendix are followed by venous engorgement, arterial compromise and subsequent gangrene.

Clinical presentation is, initially, visceral abdominal pain (due to distension of the appendix) which is poorly localized to the periumbilical region. As inflammation spreads to the parietal peritoneum the pain is sharply localized to the right iliac fossae and is exacerbated by movement or coughing. Anorexia is very frequent so that hunger should arouse suspicion of the diagnosis. Nausea and vomiting occur after the onset of abdominal pain in approximately half of patients. Change of bowel habit is not of diagnostic significance although care needs to be taken with diarrhoea which may be dominant if the inflamed appendix lies in apposition to the sigmoid colon. Urinary frequency and dysuria may occur for a similar reason when the inflamed appendix lies close to the bladder. Physical examination reveals localized tenderness over the site of the inflamed appendix. If the appendix is pelvic or retrocaecal then tenderness is elicited on pelvic or rectal examination. Localized rebound tenderness, referred rebound tenderness, or tenderness to percussion are often but not invariably present. Fever is mild but a temperature above 38.5°C should suggest perforation. Tachycardia is commensurate with the height of fever.

Diagnosis The cornerstone of diagnosis is the history and physical examination; laboratory tests and x-rays being merely ancillary.

Treatment is by appendicectomy and the only contraindication is the presence of a palpable mass 3-5 days after the onset of symptoms. In this situation, intravenous fluids and broad spectrum antibiotics are the treatment of choice. Interval appendicectomy should be performed three months later.

Appendicolysis
Surgical division of adhesions around the appendix.

Appendicostomy
Opening from the surface of the abdominal wall into the vermiform appendix performed surgically for irrigating or draining the large bowel.

Appendix (pl. appendixes, appendices)
Frequently used alone to refer to the appendix vermiformis. See also *Appendix vermiformis*

Appendix vermiformis, vermiform appendix
A redundant organ at the blind end of the caecum, 3-8 cm in length and ½ cm in diameter.

Aproctia
Congenital absence of the anus.

APUD cells (amine precursor uptake and decarboxylation cells)
The characteristics of these cells are to contain a fluorogenic amine, an amino acid decarboxylase and inhibit uptake of amine precursors. They are widespread throughout the body particularly in the gut endocrine glands. At least some are of neural crest origin. The cells contain neurosecretory granules and produce a wide range of peptide hormones. They constitute the diffuse neuro-endocrine system. Characteristic syndromes are produced in tumours (apudomas) due to excesses of particular hormones.

Arachidonic acid
see *Prostaglandin metabolism*

Arachnogastria
Prominent veins on the abdomen caused by ascites. They are noted particularly in hepatic cirrhosis.

Arbaprostil
A synthetic 15-methyl analogue of dinoprostone, a prostaglandin of the E type. It has been used orally to reduce gastric secretion in the treatment of gastric ulcer. See also *Prostaglandins*

Area nuda hepatis
More commonly called the bare area of the liver. This is the superior surface of the liver, adjacent to the diaphragm, without overlying peritoneum. Its boundaries are formed by the hepatic coronary ligament and the triangular ligaments.

Argentaffin cell
A cell showing characteristic granules produced by their ability to reduce silver nitrate to silver. They are part of the APUD system.

Argentaffinoma
A tumour of the gastroenteric tract formed from the argentaffin cells. See also *Carcinoid*

Argon laser photocoagulation
One of three types of lasers for control of upper gastrointestinal bleeding, the others being neodynium, NdYAG laser and

CO_2 laser. Argon laser photocoagulation operates in the blue green wavelength being focused onto a quartz fibre. One problem is that red blood absorbs the laser beam, which is overcome by directing a jet of gas at the bleeding point. It is very effective in oozing, but less so when there is an artery pumping in the base of the ulcer. However, mortality and the subsequent need for operation was not reduced in one clinical study. See also *Lasers*

Argyrophyl cell
A cell capable of reducing silver nitrate to silver but only in the presence of an external reducing agent. The cells are part of the APUD system.

Arsenic
Fowler's solution (arsenic trioxide) when used over long periods for psoriasis may lead to intrahepatic portal hypertension. Liver biopsy reveals portal tract fibrosis and thickened portal vein branches. Angiosarcoma is a very rare complication.

Arterial-enteric fistula
Aneurysms of the aorta and branches of the coeliac artery occasionally form fistulae into the upper gastrointestinal tract. A herald bleed is common hours or even weeks prior to a sudden cataclysmic haemorrhage. An aneurysm associated with an aortic graft with fistula formation into the duodenum is more common.

Arteriobiliary fistula
A rare condition presenting with haematobilia and due to a number of different conditions such as trauma, liver biopsy, hepatic artery aneurysm, hepatic abscess, and gallstones. Presenting features include upper gastrointestinal bleeding, associated with jaundice and biliary colic. Diagnosis is made at endoscopy with bleeding seen coming from the ampulla of Vater. Treatment is with hepatic artery embolization or ligation.

Arterio-hepatic dysplasia
An autosomal dominant condition, presenting in infancy, in which there is reduction of the number of bile ducts within the liver. It is associated with pulmonary stenosis and skeletal abnormalities.

Arteriovenous malformation(s)
see *Angiodysplasia*

Arteritis, gastrointestinal vascular involvement
This is usually, but not invariably, part of a systemic disease characterized by inflammation, often with fibrinoid necrosis of the wall of small and medium-sized arteries. Aneurysms may form, and the damaged vessels bleed or occlude leading to symptoms and infarction. Angiography is often diagnostic in polyarteritis nodosa and helps to assess the extent of the disease. See also *Polyarteritis nodosa*

Ascariasis
An infection by the roundworm *Ascaris lumbricoides*, which is found in the small intestine, causing colicky pain and diarrhoea, especially in children. On ingestion, the larvae migrate from the intestine to the lungs where they cause a pneumonitis, and then to the trachea, where they are swallowed, and finally reach the intestine, where they mature. If adult worms are present in sufficient number they may cause intestinal obstruction. (Figure 16)

Ascending colon
That part of the colon between the hepatic flexure and the caecum.

Ascites
The accumulation of serous fluid in the peritoneal cavity.
Causes There are many causes, including infections, such as tuberculosis, metastatic cancer with peritoneal seeding, portal hypertension (especially due to liver cirrhosis), hypoalbuminaemia, nephrotic

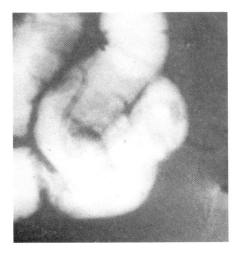

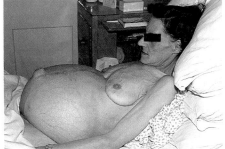

Figure 16 Ascariasis. *Ascaris lumbricoides* (round worm) seen on a barium follow-through examination of the small intestine.

syndrome, congestive cardiac failure, and protein-losing enteropathy. Rarer causes include chronic pancreatitis and bile ascites after trauma, liver biopsy, or biliary tract surgery.

Diagnosis is confirmed by ultrasound or computed tomography of the abdomen and paracentesis should always be performed. The protein concentration will determine if it is an exudate (protein greater than 30 gm/l) or transudate (protein less than 30 gm/l).

Other laboratory tests include a white cell count and differential, culture, amylase glucose, lactate dehydrogenase, culture for tuberculosis, and cytology. Peritoneoscopy is used in Europe and USA but not routinely in the UK. It is a safe, accurate method of inspecting the peritoneum, particularly when peritoneal disease is suspected. Ascites is not a diagnosis but should stimulate the physician to discover the pathological condition causing it. (Figure 17a and b) See also *Diuretics in ascites*

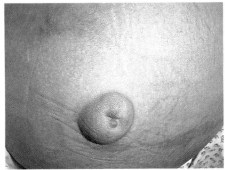

Figure 17a Ascites. A patient with tense ascites secondary to liver cirrhosis. Note the protuberant abdomen, everted umbilicus and prominent abdominal veins together with generalized muscle wasting seen in the limbs, upper arms and face. (*courtesy of Dr. A.J. Levi*).

Figure 17b Ascites. Close-up view of everted umbilicus and prominent superficial abdominal veins draining away from the umbilicus. (*courtesy of Dr. A.J. Levi*).

Ascitic fluid infusion

A form of treatment for ascites where peritoneal fluid is removed, passed through an ultrafiltration apparatus, and reinfused by an intravenous line. It is expensive and contraindicated with malignant ascites, infective ascites, and where very high protein levels can block the filter. The main complications include transient fever, intravascular fluid overload with pulmonary oedema, and intraperitoneal bleeding. See also *Ascites*

Aspartate transaminase (AST)

A mitochondrial enzyme present in liver, heart, skeletal muscle and kidney, which is released from the tissues into the blood when acute tissue damage occurs. It is useful in the diagnosis of viral hepatitis and other causes of liver cell damage. In myocardial infarction, values are raised together with a concomitant rise in creatine kinase and lactate dehydrogenase.

Aspiration biopsy cytology

A diagnostic technique of increasing use due to improvements of radiological imaging. A fine needle is placed into the lesion under ultrasound or computed tomography control. Aspirated material is examined cytologically. This technique is most commonly applied to pancreatic or hepatic malignancies.

Aspiration biopsy of pancreas

Cytological diagnosis of pancreatic cancer can be made by percutaneous fine needle aspiration. Radiological control is required either by ultrasound or computed tomography. In experienced hands the technique is relatively safe and accurate.

Aspiration, in oesophageal disorders

Both peristaltic failure of the oesophagus (achalasia) and upper oesophageal motor disorders can present with aspiration of food and fluid into the lungs, particularly at night. Pharyngeal pouches, oesophageal strictures, and cancers of the oesophagus are structural causes of this condition. The investigations of choice include barium swallow and endoscopy. See also *Oesophagus*

Aspirin

Aspirin is a useful, effective analgesic. However, it damages the gastric mucosa, causing acute erosions, ulceration and/or haemorrhage. Chronic aspirin ingestion is associated with a 2-6 fold risk of developing a peptic ulcer. Patients with a preceding history of peptic ulcer should not be prescribed this drug because bleeding may be precipitated. Aspirin ingestion entails a higher risk for gastric ulcer than duodenal ulcer. The overall risk of patients on aspirin is 0.4% per year of developing a peptic ulcer.

Asplenia

Absence of the spleen.

Asterixis

(*also known as* Flapping tremor: Liver flap) A motor disturbance marked by intermittent lapse of an assumed posture, particularly extension at the elbow and wrists. It is characteristic of hepatic coma but observed also in many other conditions, for example respiratory and renal failure.

Atresia

Congenital absence or closure of tubular organs or openings of the body which requires surgical treatment.
Bile duct atresia results in persistent jaundice and liver damage.
Duodenal atresia is often associated with Down's syndrome, but needs immediate treatment because of vomiting, epigastric distention, and lack of bowel movements. When the intestine is involved the closure can cause obstruction at any level but the ileum is most commonly affected.
Oesophageal atresia also requires surgical treatment because of symptoms which can include vomiting, cyanosis, dyspnoea and tracheo-oesophageal fistula.

Atrophic gastritis

see *Gastritis*

Atropine

An anticholinergic drug used mainly as an antispasmodic to relax smooth muscle and to dry secretions prior to gastroscopy. Side-effects may include dry mouth, blurred vision, and tachycardia. Atropine blocks the action of acetylcholine at the neuromuscular and neurosecretory junctions. See also *Anticholinergic drugs*

Auerbach's ganglion, (plexus)
(Leopold Auerbach, German anatomist, 1828-1897)
A neural plexus from the oesophagus to the anus, lying between the circular and longitudinal muscle layers. Congenital absence in Hirschsprung's disease leads to constipation and massive bowel dilatation proximal to this segment of colon. (Figure 18)

Autoantibodies
These are antibodies directed against self and may be formed in some types of liver disease. For example, in lupoid or chronic active hepatitis, autoantibodies are present against smooth muscle and nuclear cell components. IgG, IgM and IgA are often raised and in liver tissue, lymphocytes and plasma cells are prominent in portal zones and infiltrate between liver cells. In primary biliary cirrhosis antimitochondrial antibodies are present and represent a diagnostic marker of the disorder. Autoantibodies are not confined to liver disease. Antireticulin antibodies are associated with coeliac disease, antithyroid antibodies with autoimmune thyroid disease and antiparietal cell antibodies with pernicious anaemia. Autoantibodies are associated with several diseases but are not necessarily implicated in their pathogenesis, it being equally likely they are the result rather than the cause of tissue damage.

Autodigestion
After death, digestion of the stomach and surrounding structures occurs, due to release of lysosomal enzymes from dead tissues.

Autotransplantation, of pancreas
Vascularized and denervated portions of pancreas have been autotransplanted in a small number of patients undergoing subtotal or total pancreatectomy. This has improved glucose homeostasis, and, in some, prevented the inexorable development of diabetes mellitus.

Axial tomographic scanning
see *Computed tomographic scanning (CT scanning)*

Azathioprine
This is a purine analogue antimetabolite drug occasionally used as a steroid sparing agent in Crohn's disease. Its use is controversial and side-effects include bone marrow suppression, and gastrointestinal upset. In ulcerative colitis, there is no evidence of any benefit and it should not be used.

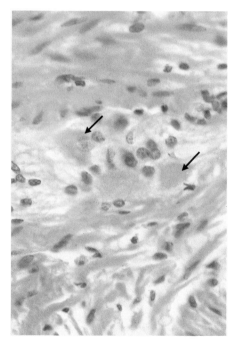

Figure 18 Auerbach's ganglion Histological section of circular muscle above and longitudinal muscle below. Auerbach's plexus with ganglion cells lies between the two muscle layers (arrowed).

Azotaemia

Azotaemia
In hepatorenal syndrome, renal failure
occurs in a patient with normal tubular
function, and chronic liver disease.
Azotaemia is often precipitated by reduced
intravascular volume caused by over-
enthusiastic diuretic treatment,
paracentesis or diarrhoea. Features of
uraemia are often absent, but the
prognosis is very grave.

B

Ba
Chemical symbol for barium. See also
Barium sulphate

Bacillus
A genus of microorganisms of the family
Bacillaceae.
Bacillus cereus is an aerobic, spore-
forming, Gram-positive bacillus that has
been implicated in several outbreaks of
food poisoning. It produces an enterotoxin
thought to be responsible for diarrhoea
and vomiting. *Bacillus paracolon*, a
microorganism, which slowly ferments
lactose is commonly found in the intestinal
flora. See also *Paracolobactrum*

Bacterial diarrhoea
see *Diarrhoea*

Bacterial infections
The whole of the gastrointestinal tract,
including liver and pancreas, may be
involved in bacterial infections which
present with varying symptoms depending
on the site. The defence mechanisms of the
gut include the intact mucosa, release of
secretions (such as saliva, containing IgA),
gastric acid, and pancreatic secretions.
The presence of a natural flora prevents
many pathogenic organisms gaining a
foothold. The immune system helps to kill
organisms seeded into the bloodstream
such as can occur after dental procedures
or colonoscopy.

Bacterial overgrowth
Bacterial overgrowth of the small bowel
occurs in the blind or stagnant loop
syndrome and presents with malabsorption of vitamin B_{12}, usually with
normal folate absorption. Steatorrhoea
occurs in one-third of patients. See also
Blind loop syndrome; *Bile-acid breath
test.*

Bacteroides
A genus of non-spore forming anaerobic
bacteria occurring as normal flora in the
mouth and large bowel. They are often
found in necrotic tissue, probably as
secondary invaders. They can be
implicated in cholangitis, septicaemia and
liver abscess. *Bacteroides fragilis* is a
pathogenic organism which may be found
in metastatic abscesses and appendicitis.

Balantidiasis
A rare, tropical infestation of the large
intestine by the parasitic protozoan
Balantidium coli. Infection occurs with
the ingestion of food or drink contaminated with cysts from the faeces of
a pig. The parasite destroys the intestinal
wall by invasion, causing ulceration and
necrosis. The main clinical feature is
diarrhoea. Recommended treatment is
tetracycline or diiodohydroxyquinoline.

Balloon tamponade
This manoeuvre is used in patients with
actively bleeding oesophageal varices,
uncontrolled by vasopressin or injection
sclerotherapy. The four lumen tube is
passed into the stomach, and the gastric
balloon inflated. Tension is maintained on
the tube to keep the gastric balloon firmly
against the gastro-oesophageal junction,
compressing the varices as they run
into the oesophagus. Inflation of the
oesophageal balloon to 30-40 mmHg to
obliterate the low pressure varices may
also be necessary (Figure 19). Bleeding
stops in 75-90% of cases. Complications
include oesophageal perforation and
aspiration pneumonia in up to 15% of
patients.

Banti's syndrome
(Guido Banti, Italian pathologist, 1852-
1925)
A disorder in which there is enlargement
and overactivity of the spleen, most
commonly caused by cirrhosis of the
liver.

Barium enema

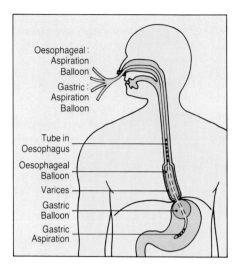

Figure 19 Balloon tamponade. Diagram showing a four lumen tube which may be passed nasally or orally under light sedation. After the tube is well into the stomach (confirmed either by aspiration of gastric contents or by x-ray) the gastric balloon is inflated with 300-400 mls of air. Firm tension is then maintained on the tube so that the gastric balloon is tight against the gastro-oesophageal junction. This may be achieved by hanging a 0.5 kg. weight over a pulley system or attaching a rubber stopper over the tube and applying traction which is maintained by firmly taping the rubber stopper to the tube. The oesophageal balloon maybe inflated to 30-40 mmHg to obliterate the bleeding oesophageal varices. Hourly gastric aspiration and continuous drainage with half-hourly oesophageal aspiration is recommended. After 24 hours the traction is released and the balloon deflated.

Barium enema
A radiological investigation to outline the anatomy and pathology of the colon. Following intubation of the rectum, barium sulphate flows to the caecum and outlines the large bowel and sometimes terminal ileum. The double contrast techniques with air afford excellent mucosal detail. Indications include suspected colonic carcinoma, inflammatory bowel disease and ischaemic or radiation strictures. (Figure 20)

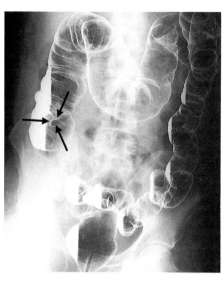

Figure 20 Barium enema. Double contrast barium enema radiograph showing the normal colon outlined with barium and air. Note the normal ileocaecal valve (arrowed).

Barium follow-through
A radiological investigation to visualize the small intestine. Barium is introduced either by nasoenteric intubation (or by ingestion) into the small intestine and serial radiographs are taken over a period of several hours. Barium follow-through is used in the diagnosis of small bowel pathology such as coeliac disease, Crohn's disease, ileocaecal tuberculosis and intestinal lymphoma. (Figure 21)

Barium meal
A radiological investigation to delineate the anatomy and pathology of the oesophagus, stomach and duodenum. Barium sulphate is swallowed under radiographic control. The outline of the oesophagus, stomach and duodenum

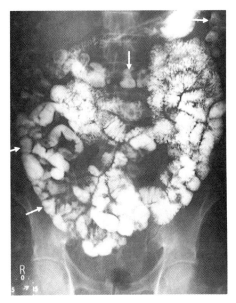

Figure 21 Barium follow-through.
Radiograph showing normal feathery pattern in the jejunum with normal ileal loops of small intestine. The colon is also partially filled (arrowed).

can be visualized and a series of radiographs is taken. Indications include suspected reflex oesophagitis (dyspepsia), achalasia, oesophageal stricture, gastric ulcer, carcinoma or duodenal ulcer. The examination is with double contrast (air and barium) and affords accurate diagnosis for upper gastrointestinal pathology. A barium meal is complementary to oesophagogastro-duodenoscopy. (Figure 22a, b and c)

Barium sulphate
A bulky, fine, white powder used as a contrast medium in the radiology of the digestive tract.

Barrett's epithelium (oesophagus)
(Norman Rupert Barrett, English surgeon, born 1903)
This is the replacement of normal squamous epithelium of the oesophagus by columnar epithelium. It occurs most commonly in patients with severe and continuous reflux oesophagitis. It may be a marker of potential malignancy and therefore some authorities recommend regular endoscopic and cytological follow-up. When first described was believed to be due to a congenitally short oesophagus.

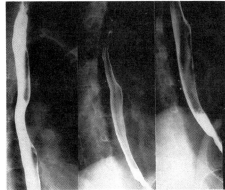

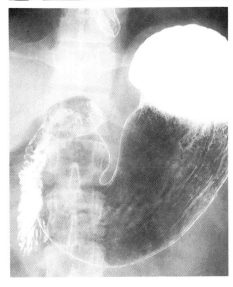

Figure 22a Barium meal. Normal oesophagus outlined with barium.
Figure 22b Barium meal. Normal stomach shown in double contrast.

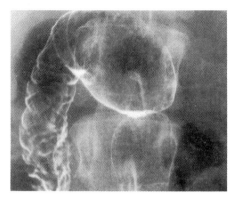

Figure 22c Barium meal. Normal duodenum. This series of radiographs represent one examination on the same patient.

Barrier, gastric mucosal
see *Mucosal barrier*

Bassen-Kornzweig disease
(Frank Albert Bassen, U.S. physician, born 1903; Albert Leon Kornzweig, U.S. physician, born 1900)
see *Abetalipoproteinaemia*

BCNU (1,3-Bis(2-chloroethyl)-1-nitrosourea: Carmustine)
An antineoplastic drug used to treat colonic carcinoma. See also *Colonic carcinoma*

Beef tapeworm
Taenia saginata infection occurs when inadequately cooked beef containing viable cysticercus larvae is ingested. On digestion of the infected meat, the cysticercus is released, the scolex evaginates and attaches to the small bowel mucosa and the worm grows up to a length of 12 to 15 feet. Clinical symptoms are due to mechanical obstruction, undernutrition and the absorption of toxic metabolites. Diagnosis depends on finding ova or proglottides in the stool. Treatment is niclosamide, four 500 mg tablets chewed in a single dose after a light meal.

Behçet's syndrome
(Halushi Behçet, Turkish dermatologist, 1889-1948)
This is an uncommon multisystem disorder of unknown pathogenesis. The pathological findings are non-specific but the main feature is a small vessel vasculitis. The diagnosis is based on clinical grounds. The major diagnostic criteria are recurrent orogenital ulceration, ocular inflammation, and skin lesions. Minor diagnostic criteria can include gastrointestinal pathology, thrombophlebitis, cardiovascular lesions, arthritis, central nervous system lesions, and a positive family history. Three major or two major and two minor criteria are required for the diagnosis. Assessment of treatment is difficult because of small numbers of patients. Corticosteroids, cytotoxic drugs, colchicine and levamisole have been used with varying success. Treatment and assessment should be conducted in large centres with specialist interest and expertise.

Belching
Eructation. The noisy release of gas from the stomach through the mouth. Air is usually swallowed with food or liquid and then released. The symptom does not imply oesophageal disease. Gas production by bacteria can occur leading to belching.

Benoxyprofen hepatotoxicity
This drug caused a serious hepatitis in the elderly. Over 60 deaths have been reported necessitating its withdrawal from use. See also *Hepatotoxicity*.

Benzimidazoles, substituted, for peptic ulcer
These are a new class of antisecretory drugs which reduce acid secretion by inhibiting a hydrogen/potassium adenosine triphosphate enzyme (ATPase) found only in gastric parietal cells. They are currently being evaluated for the treatment of duodenal ulcer and in the management of

the Zollinger-Ellison syndrome. See also *Omeprazole*

Bernstein test
This test described in 1958 is designed to establish whether a patient's symptoms of heartburn or pain are reproduced by acid perfusion of the oesophageal mucosa. A tube is placed in the oesophagus 30cm from the teeth, with a three-way stopcock allowing infusion of either normal saline or 0.1 normal hydrochloric acid.
Reproduction of the patient's symptoms by acid implies a positive test, and suggests that they are of oesophageal origin.

Beryllium poisoning
Exposure to beryllium may lead to pulmonary and hepatic granulomas.

Bethanechol (urecholine)
A cholinergic agent which has been shown to elevate the lower oesophageal sphincter pressure in normal subjects and patients with oesophageal reflux. In a study this was demonstrated to reduce the reflux of acid into the oesophagus in the treated group. Bethanechol reduces symptoms of heartburn and consequently the use of antacids. It has been reported to reduce nocturnal reflux of acid into the oesophagus using 24-hour pH monitoring. Symptoms tend to be alleviated rather than completely abolished. Bethanechol is occasionally used in the treatment of gastric retention following vagotomy.

Bezoar
A concretion of ingested material found in the stomach or bowel of man or animals. When found in man, bezoars can present serious medical problems such as epigastric pain, nausea, intestinal obstruction or upper gastrointestinal ulceration and bleeding. Diagnosis is by radiology or endoscopy. Bezoars are more common following gastrectomy with gastric stasis. Surgical management is advisable if the bezoar is large or if serious symptoms result. (Figure 23)

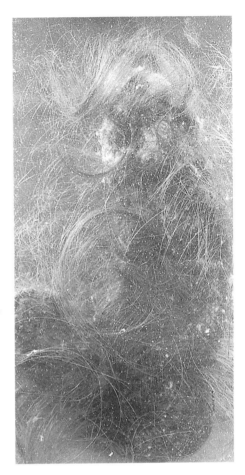

Figure 23 Bezoar. This example, comprising mats of hair, is seen in the stomach.

Bicarbonate secretion
Bicarbonate secretion has been demonstrated from oxyntic, pyloric and duodenal mucosa, which is both passive and active. In the stomach there is a pH gradient across the mucous layer so that on the mucosal surface the pH is neutral. This protects the cells from the effects of acid. The mechanism of secretion is unclear.

Bile

A complex fluid containing water, inorganic electrolytes and organic solutes such as bile acids, phospholipids, cholesterol and bilirubin. It is isosmotic with plasma and formed from hepatocytes in bile canaliculi of the liver. This process involves active transport involving ATPase and the sodium/potassium pump. Bile is then concentrated and stored in the gallbladder and ejected intermittently into the duodenum, via the common bile duct. With the entry of food into the duodenum, the gallbladder contracts mainly under the stimulus of hormonal factors. Bile is able to emulsify fat which renders it more easily digested. In the terminal ileum bile salts are reabsorbed under the influence of the enterohepatic circulation and then returned to the liver. The formation of bile is essential for excreting certain waste products, such as bilirubin, as well as the excretion of many drugs and toxins. It is essential for normal lipid absorption and is a major source of cholesterol excretion. Bile may play an important role in the delivery of IgA to the gastrointestinal tract. Bile stasis and failure of secretion (cholestasis) occur which may lead to ascending cholangitis, septicaemia, and the formation of gallstones.

Bile acids are the organic acids, mainly present as the bile salts sodium glycocholate and sodium taurocholate. Bile acids also include cholic acid, deoxycholic acid, glycocholic acid, and taurocholic acid. They are capable of emulsifying fats.

Bile-acid breath test

This is a test for bacterial overgrowth of the small intestine, which is influenced by ileal dysfunction. Conjugated ^{14}C-glycine and bile acid is normally absorbed at the terminal ileum intact. However, exposure to large amounts of bacteria in the small intestine results in the premature release of ^{14}C-glycine which is metabolized to $^{14}CO_2$ and excreted and measured in the breath. See also *Bacterial overgrowth.*

Bile canaliculi

These channels within the liver are the starting point of bile excretion. They have no walls and are channels between adjacent liver cells. The latter are covered by microvilli at that site and their cytoskeleton is reinforced by microfilaments. The canaliculi drain directly into terminal bile ducts carrying bile towards the gallbladder.

Bile ducts

These ducts convey bile from the liver to the duodenum via the gallbladder and the common bile duct. Bile from canaliculi drains into the smallest thin-walled terminal bile ducts which combine to form larger ducts draining into the right and left hepatic ducts which ultimately terminate in the common hepatic duct. The cystic duct, leading from the gallbladder, joins the common hepatic duct to form the common bile duct which drains into the duodenum by way of the ampulla of Vater. The anatomy of the bile ducts is outlined radiologically at endoscopic retrograde cholangiopancreatography (ERCP). Abnormally dilated ducts may be cannulated percutaneously. (Figure 24)

Bile peritonitis

see *Peritonitis, bile (biliary)*

Bile pigment-calcium stones

see *Gallstones*

Bile reflux

Duodenogastric reflux of bile from the duodenum into the stomach is commonly observed at endoscopy. It is present in normal individuals, in patients with peptic ulcer disease, and following gastric surgery. Reflux of bile is caused by retrograde peristalsis, and is thought to produce symptoms of nausea, vomiting bile, heartburn, and anorexia. After gastric surgery bile reflux is commonly observed endoscopically but seldom produces symptoms. If symptoms occur, dietary manipulation and oral metoclopramide are

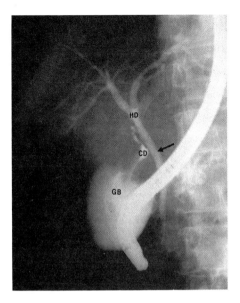

Figure 24 Bile ducts. ERCP showing the gallbladder filled with contrast medium (GB). The cystic duct (CD) joins the common hepatic duct (HD) to form the common bile duct (arrowed). The hepatic ducts form a branching pattern draining bile from the periphery of the liver joining to form the right and left hepatic duct.

often successful. Recalcitrant symptoms occur in a very small number of patients when diversion operations, such as a Roux-en-Y conversion, are required.

Pancreatic reflux is reflux of bile into the pancreatic duct following obstruction of the ampulla of Vater by a gallstone. This has been proposed as a mechanism for the development of acute pancreatitis.
See also *Pancreatitis, acute*

Biliary atresia, extra-hepatic
This is a congenital malformation of the biliary tree, presenting in the neonatal period with obstructive jaundice and pruritus, which is progressive and unremitting. Death is usually due to intercurrent infections, liver cell failure, or to bleeding from oesophageal varices.

Recently liver transplantation has been attempted with varying success.

Biliary cirrhosis
see *Cirrhosis*

Biliary colic
This typically consists of upper abdominal or right hypochondrial severe steady pain (not intermittent as suggested by the word colic) gradually increasing over an hour and lasting several hours with gradual remission. The pain often radiates to the back, a symptom helping in the diagnosis. Vomiting commonly occurs. The symptoms are due to obstruction of the common bile duct or gallbladder by a stone. Attacks are unpredictable, occurring at varying intervals, and may be mistaken for gastric, duodenal or pancreatic pathology.

Biliary cystadenoma
A rare benign tumour of the liver of bile duct origin, predominantly in the elderly. Patients complain of abdominal discomfort and a mass may be felt. The cysts are usually solitary and are lined by a single layer of cuboidal/columnar "biliary" epithelium.

Biliary fistulae
These are abnormal communications between the biliary tree and usually the gastrointestinal tract. Common causes include procedures such as cholecystotomy, transhepatic biliary drainage or T-tube choledochotomy. There is usually a long history of biliary disease, and the fistula may be symptomless. Approximately 30% of patients have jaundice. Pain or cholangitis may occur, with diarrhoea and weight loss. Management requires drainage of the common bile duct, endoscopically or by surgery.

Biliary tract
The anatomy includes the right and left hepatic ducts emerging from the right and

Bilious

left lobes of the liver at the porta hepatis. This merging forms the common hepatic duct which is joined by the cystic duct to form the common bile duct, draining into the duodenum through the ampulla of Vater. The gallbladder joins the cystic duct at its narrow neck. (Figure 25)

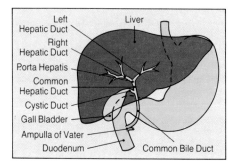

Figure 25   Biliary tract.

Bilious

A lay term which includes symptoms of nausea, abdominal discomfort, flatulence and constipation previously ascribed to excess bile secretion. *Bilious vomiting* is the vomiting of bile-stained fluid.

Bilirubin

A bile pigment formed by the normal breakdown of haemoglobin from red blood cells. Excess production, or reduced excretion of bilirubin leads to jaundice, an abnormal staining of tissues and body fluids seen best in the sclera. Bilirubin is insoluble in water in the unconjugated form, measured as indirect bilirubin, and is not excreted in the urine. It is elevated in haemolytic conditions and the uncommon disorders of bilirubin metabolism. Conjugated bilirubin is soluble, appears in the urine, and is elevated in cholestasis. In the laboratory it is measured as direct bilirubin. The majority of bilirubin circulates in the plasma tightly bound to albumin, is taken up by liver cells and conjugated to bilirubin diglucuronide. This soluble product is secreted into the bile

canaliculi, collects in the gallbladder and is excreted in faeces. Normal serum bilirubin values are less than 0.8 mg/100 mls. If levels rise to 1.5 mg/100 mls jaundice is detectable clinically. Bilirubin is not found in the urine of healthy individuals.

Bilirubinuria
Bilirubin present in the urine.

Biliuria
Bile pigments present in the urine.

Biliverdin
The initial green bile pigment obtained from the breakdown of haemoglobin.

Billroth I
(Christian Albert Theodor Billroth, German surgeon, 1829-1894)
Billroth I is a classical operation for gastric ulcer disease which was used extensively in the 1950s and 1960s. A partial gastrectomy is performed with the ulcer included in the resected specimen. The gastric portion of the remaining part is partially closed, leaving a stoma which is joined directly to the resected part of the duodenum. Recurrence of ulcer is less than 1% for this operation. (Figure 26)

Billroth II
A partial gastrectomy is performed as for the Billroth I operation. The duodenal stump is then closed and the first loop of the jejunum is anastomosed to the gastric stoma forming a gastroenterostomy. The blind ending afferent loop is made as short as possible and leads to the enterostomy from where the efferent loop drains. There are now more than 40 modifications of this operation. (Figure 27)

Biopsy capsule
A small metal device attached to a thin, hollow, long plastic tube. It is spring-loaded and passed by mouth or an endoscope into the small intestine, where it is 'fired' by negative pressure from a 20ml syringe ('popping' the syringe).

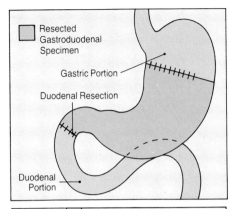

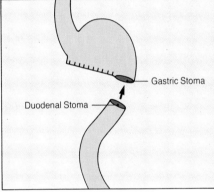

Figure 26 Billroth I. Diagram of Billroth I operation showing resected gastroduodenal specimen and union of the gastric stoma to the duodenal stoma.

Biopsies from the mucosa are examined microscopically. Several different types of biopsy capsules are available, for example, Crosby capsule and Watson capsule.

Bisacodyl
A cathartic laxative active orally and rectally, leading to reflex movement of the large bowel and evacuation. It is useful in preparation for radiological procedures and endoscopy. Tablets act within 10 to 12 hours while suppositories are effective within one hour. Side-effects are restricted to cramping abdominal pain.

Stimulant laxatives such as bisacodyl are contraindicated with intestinal obstruction. Prolonged use should be avoided because of possible complications of hypokalaemia and an atonic non-functioning colon.

Bismuth
Tri-potassium di-citrato bismuthate. Bismuth salts have previously been used for the treatment of syphilis. Recently tri-potassium di-citrato bismuthate, a bismuth chelate, has been used for the treatment of both gastric and duodenal ulcers. The mechanism of action is uncertain, but it is believed to coat the ulcer and promote healing. It is therefore administered on an empty stomach to prevent its adherence to food. It is available as a pungent aromatic liquid and in tablet form. Tri-potassium di-citrato bismuthate has been shown to heal peptic ulcers effectively. A recent paper has shown it to be effective against histologically proven gastritis with symptomatic relief, and histological improvement.

Bismuth poisoning
(*also known as* Bismuthism: Bismuthosis)
Chronic poisoning is characterized by anuria, stomatitis, dermatitis and diarrhoea.

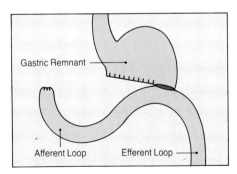

Figure 27 Billroth II. Diagram of Billroth II operation showing gastric remnant, blind ending afferent duodenal loop and efferent jejunal drainage limb.

Bleeding

Encephalopathy is a rare side-effect previously seen only with intramuscular administration for syphilis.

Bleeding

See *Gastrointestinal bleeding (haemorrhage): Oesophageal varices*

Blennorrhagia

Excess mucous discharge.

Blind loop syndrome

(*also known as* Stagnant loop: Stasis syndrome) The development of malabsorption in a patient with bacterial overgrowth within the small bowel. Small numbers of Gram-positive aerobes or facultative anaerobes inhabit the normal small intestine. Any abnormality resulting in local stasis will allow a significant proliferation of these organisms and the possibility of developing malabsorption. Such conditions predisposing to blind loop syndrome include abdominal surgery, structural abnormalities (for example, Crohn's disease or radiation enteritis), motor disorders (for example, scleroderma), or achlorhydria.

Clinical features vary greatly from no symptoms to anaemia, steatorrhoea, weight loss, abdominal pain and swelling. Anaemia is caused by vitamin B_{12} deficiency and neurological symptoms identical to those of pernicious anaemia may develop.

Diagnosis is suggested by a macrocytic anaemia, and vitamin B_{12} deficiency with normal or raised serum folate levels. Small bowel enemas will outline the anatomy, and properly collected and appropriately cultured proximal small bowel aspirate confirms the diagnosis. A ^{14}C xylose breath test proves to be a sensitive and specific test to diagnose the presence of bacterial overgrowth and has superseded the ^{14}C-glycine test.

Treatment by antibiotics reduces or eliminates bacterial overgrowth. Tetracycline will provide clinical improvement within one week in 50% of patients. If there is no response other antibiotics are chosen. Vitamin B_{12} and nutritional supplementation aid recovery.

Bloat

Gaseous distention of the abdomen.

Blumberg's sign

(Jacob Moritz Blumberg, German gynaecologist and surgeon, 1873-1955) Increased pain on rapid release of steady pressure over the abdomen, which correlates with peritonism and peritonitis. See also *Rebound tenderness.*

Bochdalek's hernia

(Vincenz Alexander Bochdalek, Czech anatomist, 1801-1883) see *Hernia*

Bolus

A soft rounded mass of chewed food in preparation for swallowing.

Bolus obstruction

Obstruction of the oesophagus by a bolus of food, due either to incomplete chewing, or to a mechanical narrowing of the oesophagus. Symptoms include salivation, and complete inability to swallow solids or liquids, together with retrosternal discomfort. Treatment is by removal at oesophagoscopy, and dilatation of the oesophagus.

Bombesin

A peptide present in the skin of certain frogs, which on infusion into animals leads to smooth muscle contraction, gastric and pancreatic secretion, and the release of gastrin. Bombesin-like biologically active substances have been found in gastrointestinal tissues of man, and are potent inhibitors of human gastric emptying. There are no known human diseases associated with abnormal secretion of this peptide.

Borborygmi

Gurgling noises caused by the movement of gas and fluid through the intestine.

Botulism

Food poisoning caused by a neurotoxin (botulin) produced by *Clostridium botulinum* in improperly canned or preserved foods. There are seven antigenically distinct forms of toxins (A to G). Toxins A, B and E are most frequently implicated in human disease.

Clinical symptoms include vomiting, nausea and neurological symptoms of which the commonest is diplopia, blurred vision and photophobia. Progressive descending paralysis can occur and when the muscles of respiration are impaired ventilatory assistance may be required. Symptoms usually develop 12 to 36 hours after ingestion.

Treatment A trivalent antitoxin to A, B and E is available and should be used if the diagnosis is suspected. Mortality is approximately 10%, death commonly being due to respiratory failure and pneumonia. See also *Food poisoning*.

Bougie

A cylindrical, often flexible instrument, that is inserted into the oesophagus or rectum, in order to dilate a stricture or narrowing of that organ. (Figure 28)

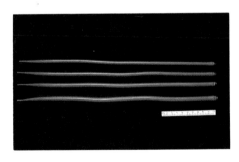

Figure 28 Bougies. Illustration of four graduated, flexible mercury-filled Pilling bougies. Note the length and soft, flexible, thin tips.

Bougienage

This procedure is performed only for histologically confirmed benign oesophageal strictures. After an overnight fast the procedure is explained to the patient who is then made comfortable. Graduated bougies of increasing size are passed into the oesophagus and gentle dilatation performed. Usually the passage of three or four bougies is required for adequate dilatation.

Bowel

see *Intestine*

Bran

The epidermis or outer covering of cereal grains. It is an important constituent of the diet providing bulk for the stool, treatment for constipation, and a probable reduction in the incidence of colorectal cancer. Highly processed foods such as white bread have most of the bran removed. Addition of bran to the highly processed Western diet avoids constipation and may reduce the risk of colorectal cancer.

Breast milk jaundice

see *Jaundice*

Breath test

A test used to diagnose bacterial overgrowth. See also *Tests*

Bromocriptine in hepatic encephalopathy

Bromocriptine causes prolonged stimulation of dopamine receptors. It also causes clinical and electroencephalogram (EEG) improvement in patients with chronic stable hepatic encephalopathy.

Bromsulphalein test

An obsolete test of liver function where a dye, bromsulphalein, is rapidly removed by the liver and excreted into the bile. Occasionally, fatal reactions have occurred bringing the test into disrepute.

Brucellosis

An infection caused by *Brucella* organisms and characterized by generalized non-specific symptoms such as fever, sweats, weakness and malaise. There is a large animal reservoir of *Brucella* organisms of which *Brucella abortus* may cause hepatic granulomas and *Brucella suis* may lead to hepatic suppuration. Liver biopsy usually shows a non-specific reactive hepatitis. Ill-formed granulomas are often a histological feature.

Bruit de clapotement

A splashing sound indicating distension of the stomach when pressure is applied to the wall of the abdomen. See also *Succussion splash*

Brunner's glands

(Johann Conrad Brunner, Swiss anatomist, 1653-1727)
Branched acinar glands containing mucous and serous secretory cells present in the submucosa of the duodenum. The secretion from Brunner's glands is rich in bicarbonate and mucus, and protects the proximal duodenum from acid-pepsin digestion.

Brushing

At endoscopy, samples of epithelial cells may be obtained by brushing the surface mucosa. These cells are fixed on slides and examined cytologically. Brushing is useful for the diagnosis of gastric and oesophageal neoplasms. Candidiasis may also be confirmed by brushing.

Buccoglossopharyngitis sicca

Dryness of the mouth, tongue and pharynx. See also *Sjögren's syndrome*

Bud

see *Liver bud: Taste bud*

Budd-Chiari syndrome (disease)

(George Budd, English physician, 1808-1882; Hans Chiari, Austrian pathologist, 1851-1916)

A rare syndrome due to obstruction of the inferior vena cava and hepatic vein which leads to ascites and hepatomegaly.

Causes of the obstruction are tumour, thrombosis and membranous obstruction of the vena cava. Presentation includes abdominal pain in about 50%, abdominal swelling due to ascites in 95%, and tender hepatomegaly. Splenomegaly and jaundice are only seen in 30% of patients.

Diagnosis is confirmed by ^{99}Tc liver scan, showing an enlarged caudate lobe. An inferior vena cava gram may reveal the level of the blockage. Liver biopsy shows centrilobular necrosis, hepatic congestion and eventually fibrosis.

Management is by anticoagulation. Underlying conditions such as tumour, polycythaemia, haemoglobinopathy and antithrombin III deficiency should be investigated. Oral contraceptives should be excluded as a cause. (Figure 29a and b)

Bulb, duodenal

see *Duodenum*

Bulb, gustatory

see *Taste bud*

Bulimarexia

Vomiting following food cramming and overeating.

Bulimia

Abnormal increase in hunger and, consequently, overeating. It is a common intermittent symptom of anorexia nervosa or may be due to lesions of the hypothalamus.

Bulkage

(*also known as* Bulking agent) Material that will increase the bulk of the intestinal contents and as a result stimulate peristalsis.

Burr cells

(*also known as* Spur cells) These are red blood cells with marked thorny projections, occurring in advanced liver

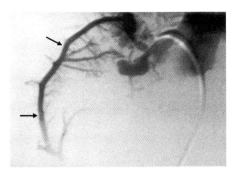

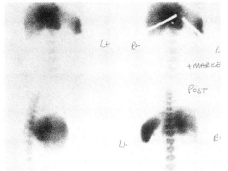

Bypass operations

Gastric Gastrojejunostomy in which the stomach is divided high on the body, while the proximal end is joined to a loop of jejunum. See also *Gastrojejunostomy Intestinal.* Resection of a part of the intestine, with anastomosis of the proximal to the distal portion, as in jejunoileostomy.

Jejunal Surgical anastomosis of the proximal part of the jejunum to the distal part of the ileum, bypassing most of the absorptive surface of the small bowel. This operation used to be performed for obesity but is associated with significant malabsorption of essential vitamins and minerals. Consequently fewer of these operations are now performed. See also *Gastroplasty*; *Jejunoileal bypass*

Figure 29a Budd-Chiari syndrome.
Hepatic vein digital subtraction angiograph showing the tip of the catheter at the origin of the hepatic vein. There is complete obstruction without any filling of the hepatic venous radicles. The arrows show collateral filling of a vessel probably near the hepatic capsule.
Figure 29b Budd-Chiari syndrome. A technetium liver scan showing a prominent caudate lobe with reduced uptake in the rest of the liver. Increased bone marrow uptake indicates poor hepatic function. The spleen is enlarged.

disease, especially in alcoholics, and in patients with severe anaemia and haemolysis. Their presence implies a poor prognosis.

Byler's disease
see *Cholestasis*

C

Caecal volvulus
This condition occurs when the caecum is attached to a long mesentery and rotates about itself leading to impairment of the blood supply. Symptoms include right-sided abdominal pain and a short history of constipation. See also *Volvulus*

Caecectomy
Surgical removal of the caecum.

Caecolopexy (caecolofixation)
An operation to stabilize the caecum and ascending colon.

Caecostomy
An operation where the caecum is opened and drained to decompress the intestine, usually when the colon is obstructed or injured.

Caecum
A blind-ending pouch into which open the ileocaecal valve and appendix. It is the first part of the large intestine and is continuous with the ascending colon.

Calcium absorption
Calcium is absorbed from the proximal small intestine in the ionized form. Calcium is transported against an electrical and chemical gradient by means of a carrier protein found in the surface membrane of the small intestine. Vitamin D plays a major role in facilitating calcium absorption. Parathyroid hormone (PTH) and a calcium deficient state also increases absorption of calcium but to a lesser extent. Local binding to gut contents reduces calcium absorption, particularly if there is a high intraluminal fatty acid content due to fat malabsorption.

Calcium carbonate
An antacid which converts hydrochloric acid to soluble calcium chloride. Excess calcium absorption may lead to hypercalcaemia, therefore calcium carbonate is not appropriate long-term antacid therapy.

Calculus
A stone, or abnormal concretion occurring within the body, usually composed of minerals. For example, gallstones (biliary calculi) form within the gallbladder or biliary tree and are composed of a variable mixture of cholesterol, calcium salts and bile pigments, depending on the composition of bile. Pure pigment or cholesterol stones can occur. Gallstones present in the intrahepatic bile ducts and are called hepatic calculi. Pancreatic calculi found within the pancreatic duct are predominantly composed of calcium carbonate. Calculi within the intestine are termed enteroliths.

Campylobacter fetus
(*formerly known as Vibrio fetus*)
Campylobacter fetus consists of three subspecies, namely *fetus*, *intestinalis* and *jejuni*. All three are well documented animal pathogens while the latter is most frequently implicated in human disease and is a leading cause of diarrhoea.

Epidemiology Campylobacter fetus subspecies *jejuni* is the leading cause of bacterial gastroenteritis in the Western world, being isolated in 5% of patients with diarrhoea. The most common route of transmission to humans is from infected animals or foodstuffs for example, milk, raw eggs and meat. The incubation period is usually 12-72 hours, but may extend to ten days.

Clinical features The clinical spectrum of illness varies from severe diarrhoea to asymptomatic excretion. However, diarrhoea and fever occur in 90%, abdominal pain in 70% and bloody stools in 50% of patients. Other symptoms include headache, backache, myalgias, malaise, vomiting and anorexia. The illness rarely exceeds 14 days, but relapses are common.

Diagnosis is confirmed by stool culture and faecal leucocytes are commonly present in the stool, indicating intestinal inflammation.

Treatment is indicated with erythro-mycin 250-500mg. four times per day, for seven days. This treatment, if instituted early, can reduce the duration of illness.

Campylobacter pylori
This bacterium was first isolated in 1982 and in man is found chiefly on the gastric mucosa. It is a motile Gram-negative spiral rod with four to six unipolar flagellae. It requires three to five days in moist conditions, in reduced oxygen tension at 37°C for optimal growth on selective media. It is associated with histological gastritis, gastric and duodenal ulceration. Evidence is accruing that *Campylobacter pylori* is a likely cause of antral type B gastritis. (Figure 30 a and b)

Canada-Cronkhite syndrome
(Wilma Jeanne Canada, U.S. physician; Leonard W. Cronkhite, Jr, U.S. physician, born 1919)
This is a syndrome of familial intestinal polyposis combined with ectodermal defects such as alopecia, increased skin pigmentation or nail atrophy.

Canaliculus (canaliculi)
see *Biliary tract*

Cancer
see *Carcinoma: specific names, organs and regions*

Candidiasis
An infection by a fungus of the *Candida* genus. The mouth is a common site for this infection, presenting as small white adherent plaques and is often associated with either immunosuppression or concurrent antibiotic treatment. Oesophageal candidiasis is a rare condition. *Candida* infections commonly termed 'thrush' or monilia, may also affect moist areas of skin, the respiratory and genitourinary tracts. *Candida albicans* is the commonest subclass.

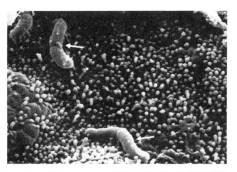

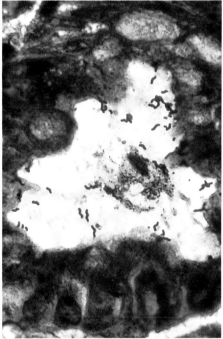

Figure 30a *Campylobacter pylori*.
Scanning electromicrograph showing spiral-shaped *Campylobacter pylori* (arrowed) lying adjacent to the gastric epithelium.
Figure 30b *Campylobacter pylori*.
Campylobacter pylori organisms in the gastric pit. (Warthin-Starry stain x 400).

Diagnosis is made on barium swallow or at gastroscopy where brushings from the oesophagus are sent for microscopy and culture. It may also be a feature of AIDS infection. In immunosuppressed patients, systemic candidiasis is a serious and life-threatening situation.

Treatment for oral candidiasis is with nystatin solution, or amphotericin lozenges. Candidiasis of the oesophagus is often treated with ketoconazole, while systemic candidiasis requires systemic amphotericin. (Figure 31)

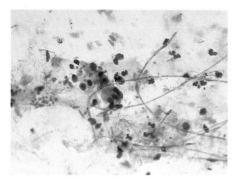

Figure 31 **Candidiasis**. The hyphae of *Candida* are easily seen in this oesophageal cytology preparation. (Papanicolau stain x 400).

Caput medusae

A network of superficial veins around the umbilicus seen in patients with cirrhosis of the liver.

Carbenoxolone

A drug that promotes healing of gastric ulcers, but has now been superseded by H_2 antagonists. The main side-effects are retention of salt and water leading to weight gain, oedema, confusion (especially in the elderly), hypertension, and hypokalaemia. These side-effects are related to its aldosterone-like activity. The mode of action is unknown but a postulated mechanism is coating of the ulcer to promote healing.

Carbohydrate

Carbohydrates contain carbon, hydrogen and oxygen, and the carbohydrate constituents in the human diet are starch, sucrose and lactose. They form an important energy source, being broken down in the body to form glucose.

Carcino-embryonic antigen (CEA)

This is an oncofetal antigen normally absent in adults but found to be elevated in patients with certain carcinomas. Initially it was thought to be specific for colorectal cancer. It is usually absent in early (Dukes A + B) colonic cancer and is no longer used as a screening test. It more reliably detects post-surgical recurrence of colonic carcinoma and may be an indicator of prognosis.

Carcinoid

A term designed to reflect the slow growth (carcinoma-like) of tumours derived from the endocrine cells of the gastrointestinal tract. They are tumours of the APUD cells and are characterized by histochemical staining for specific neurosecretory granules and by argentaffin and argyrophil techniques.

Carcinoid syndrome

This is a complex of clinical symptoms and signs due to release of biologically active chemicals from carcinoid tumours. The primary tumours arise most commonly from the appendix or the small intestine but may arise from the stomach, pancreas, common bile duct, colon or bronchial tree. These tumours are unique in possessing enterochromaffin (argentaffin) cells which have characteristic chemical and biochemical features. Development of the carcinoid syndrome usually implies extensive metastasis of tumours to the liver. (Figure 32 a and b)

Symptoms Clinical symptoms include diarrhoea, abdominal pain or cramp, episodic flushing, telangiectasia, cyanosis, wheezing and pulmonary and tricuspid valve lesions. The symptoms are due to

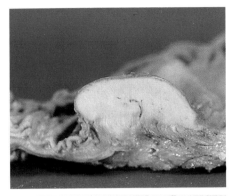

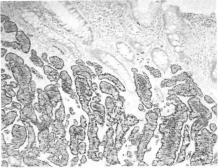

Figure 32a Carcinoid syndrome. The cut surface of a carcinoid tumour of the ileum.
Figure 32b Carcinoid syndrome. A carcinoid tumour showing the characteristic black/brown neurosecretory granules around the rim of the nests of the tumour cells. (Grimelius stain x 63).

the production or storage of 5-hydroxy-tryptamine by the tumours. This is metabolized to 5-hydroxyindoleacetic acid (5HIAA) the detection of which forms the basis of a diagnostic test on patients' urine samples. Partial surgical resection may be beneficial in patients with metastases confined to a single lobe of the liver.

Treatment Drug treatment includes cyproheptadine and serotonin antagonists which reduce flushing. Corticosteroids are particularly useful for bronchial carcinoids, while methyldopa reduces

diarrhoea in patients with gastric carcinoid syndrome. Codeine phosphate, methysergide, and perphenazine act to prevent diarrhoea. Advanced hepatic metastases may be treated with chemotherapy, or arterial embolization.

Prognosis Despite metastatic spread of this tumour, prognosis is reasonably good, particularly with patients having ileal or appendiceal carcinoids. The latter tend to present early due to acute appendicitis. Most patients survive five to ten years from diagnosis.

Table 4 Principle manifestations of carcinoid syndrome

Vasomotor disturbances
Hepatomegaly
Intestinal hypermotility
Bronchoconstriction
Cardiac features:
  endocardial fibrosis;
  valvular deformity
Absence of hypertension
Prolonged clinical course

Carcinoma

A malignant tumour of epithelial origin. Carcinoma may arise directly from non-neoplastic epithelium or from a previously existing benign epithelial tumour. It is characterized by sheets or masses of dividing tumour cells and an accompanying stroma. Carcinomas are capable of autonomous growth and if they remain untreated, cause death by local growth or an ability to metastasize. There are many special types characteristic of particular sites but the majority fall within the two classes of squamous carcinoma and adenocarcinoma named according to the type of epithelium from which they originate.

Carcinomatosis
The presence of multiple deposits of carcinoma at sites distant from the origin of the malignancy.

Carcinosarcoma, oesophageal
see *Oesophageal carcinosarcoma*

Cardia
That part of the stomach which abuts the oesophagus and contains no parietal or chief cells.

Cardiospasm
Achalasia of the oesophagus. See also *Achalasia*

Caroli's disease
(Jacques Caroli, French physician, born 1902)
A congenital disorder of the intrahepatic bile ducts comprising multiple saccular dilatations. Intrahepatic stone formation, cholangitis, or complications of portal hypertension lead to symptoms between the ages of 20 and 50 years. It is a variant of polycystic disease and there is associated hepatic fibrosis and medullary sponge disease of the kidneys in some patients. Antibiotic treatment of cholangitis and surgical removal of the stones may be helpful. Death usually occurs from recurrent attacks of cholangitis.

Cathartic
A purgative or cleansing agent causing bowel evacuation by increasing stool bulk and stimulating peristalsis. See also *Laxative*

Cathartic colon
see *Laxative abuse*

CCK
see *Cholecystokinin*

Cestodes
see *Tapeworms*

Chagas' disease
(Carlos Chagas, Brazilian physician, 1879-1934)
A disease confined to South and Central America due to *Trypanosoma cruzi*. There are two forms:
An acute illness, usually occurring in children, with fever and massive oedema, which lasts up to thirty days.
A chronic illness, with arrhythmias and congestive cardiac failure. The oesophagus is also affected, leading to gross dilatation, and a history similar to achalasia. Megacolon may also occur.

Charcot's intermittent biliary fever
(Jean Martin Charcot, French neurologist, 1825-1893)
Intermittent high fever with rigors associated with partial obstruction of the common bile duct by either a ball valve calculus or traumatic stricture. The triad of abdominal pain, jaundice and chills, indicates ascending cholangitis. See also *Cholangitis*

Chenodeoxycholic acid (CDCA)
A primary bile acid shown to be effective in dissolving gallstones. Chenodeoxycholic acid lowers biliary cholesterol by reducing liver synthesis and biliary cholesterol secretion. However, it is only effective with small (less than 1cm) radiolucent stones in a functioning gallbladder. Stone dissolution takes from 6 to 24 months, depending on size and number of stones. Recurrence of stone formation after discontinuing treatment is common. Side-effects of treatment include diarrhoea, nausea, vomiting, and liver dysfunction. See also *Ursodeoxycholic acid*

Chief cells
(*also known as* Peptic cells) Pepsin secreting cells of the gastric mucosa.

Child's classification of cirrhosis
(Charles G. Child, U.S. surgeon, born 1908)
This is the most widely used prognostic

guide in liver failure, devised by C.G. Child. The classification assesses jaundice, ascites, serum albumin, hepatic encephalopathy and nutrition.

Cholangioadenoma
This rare benign neoplastic polyp arising from the bile duct comprises a dysplastic biliary epithelium on a connective tissue stalk.

Cholangiocarcinoma
This is a malignant tumour of bile duct epithelium. It may arise from the small peripheral ducts within the liver or from larger ducts near the porta hepatis. The former has a worse prognosis as it presents late, often when metastases are already present. The latter present early due to obstructive jaundice. Characteristically the tumour forms a tough, fibrous scirrhous mass. Histologically, the common pattern is tubular, though some may be indistinguishable from hepatocellular carcinomas.

Cholangioenterostomy
Anastomosis of a bile duct to the intestine.

Cholangiography
Radiological examination of the bile ducts used to demonstrate pathology. These include:
Intravenous cholangiography, which is performed by intravenous injection of contrast material to outline the bile ducts.

Percutaneous transhepatic cholangiography (PTC), which is performed by direct injection of radio-opaque material into the bile ducts.
Operative cholangiography, which is accomplished at operation by direct cannulation of the common bile duct with injection of contrast material.
Endoscopic retrograde cholangiopancreatography (ERCP), which is brought about by cannulation of the ampulla of Vater at upper gastrointestinal endoscopy.
See also *Endoscopic retrograde cholangiopancreatography: Intravenous cholangiography: Percutaneous transhepatic cholangiography*

Cholangioma
see *Cholangioadenoma*

Cholangiopancreatography, endoscopic retrograde
see *Endoscopic retrograde cholangiopancreatography*

Cholangitis
Inflammation of bile ducts usually associated with partial biliary obstruction due to gallstones, biliary strictures, sclerosing cholangitis or, rarely, neoplastic biliary obstruction.
Clinical features Symptoms include intermittent fever (95% of patients), rigors, sweating, right upper quadrant abdominal pain (90% of patients), vomiting, pruritis, and jaundice. The stools may become pale and urine dark. Common·

Table 5 Criteria for Child-Turcotte classification

Group	A	B	C
Serum bilirubin (mg%)	Below 2.0	2.0-3.0	Over 3.0
Serum albumin (g%)	Over 3.5	3.0-5.0	Under 3.0
Ascites	None	Easily controlled	Poorly controlled
Hepatic encephalopathy	None	Minimal	Advanced (coma)
Nutrition	Excellent	Reduced	Poor (wasting)

Cholecalciferol

pathological bacteria include *Escherichia coli, Bacteroides, Klebsiella, Proteus*, and other intestinal flora. Obstructive liver function tests with a raised serum alkaline phosphatase and raised conjugated bilirubin support the diagnosis.

Differential diagnosis includes the cholestatic phase of viral hepatitis, drug jaundice, or a pancreatic malignancy. Cholangiography or laparoscopy may assist in making the correct diagnosis. Possible complications of cholangitis include septicaemic shock and liver abscess formation.

Treatment includes urgent relief of the biliary obstruction, plus antibiotics. Biliary obstruction from choledocholithiasis may be relieved by endoscopic sphincterotomy from below or by the insertion of a T-tube. Both procedures may lead to prompt resolution of symptoms. The antibiotics of choice include cefuroxime and ampicillin for mild cases, or mezlocillin, metronidazole, and gentamicin for more severe cases. See also *Choledocholithiasis*

Cholecalciferol
see *Vitamin D*

Cholecyst
see *Gallbladder*

Cholecystectomy
Surgical removal of the gallbladder. This is required in the management of acute cholecystitis and cholelithiasis. With inflammatory disease there is debate as to the timing of the operation. Early cholecystectomy is undertaken within two or three days of an acute attack. Interval cholecystectomy is performed after a period of four to six weeks, when the patient has fully recovered. If concurrent medical illness is present then late cholecystectomy is appropriate. Current opinion favours early cholecystectomy with a reduction in hospitalization time, cost, and more rapid recovery. Morbidity and mortality rates are similar for both operations (Table 6).

Table 6 Consolidated results of four controlled trials comparing early and interval cholecystectomy for acute cholecystitis

	Timing of Cholecystectomy	
	Early	Interval
No. of patients	215	192
Deaths	0	5
Duct injuries	0	0
Total mean hospital stay days	10.9	20.1
Failure of regimen	N/A	19%

* Failure of regimen means surgery was required for progressive acute disease

Cholecystenterostomy
(*also known as* Cholecystoenterostomy)
This is a surgical procedure joining the gallbladder with the small intestine to allow bile to drain from the liver to the intestine. It is usually performed to bypass a malignancy.

Cholecystitis
Inflammation of the gallbladder which may take two main forms:
Acute cholecystitis 90% of these patients have gallstones with obstruction of the cystic duct. Bacteria, including coliform organisms, *Streptococcus, Staphylococcus, Clostridium, Salmonella* and anaerobic organisms, especially *Bacteroides*, are isolated in half of the patients.

Clinical features are severe right upper quadrant steady pain radiating to the back, headache, nausea, vomiting and fever. Abdominal examination reveals rebound tenderness in the right upper quadrant with a positive Murphy's sign. An inflamed distended gallbladder may be palpable or visible but jaundice is usually absent. Investigations should include plain x-ray of the abdomen, biliary scintigraphy (HIDA-scan, if available) and ultrasound of the gallbladder.

Management is by cholecystectomy covered with antibiotics. The excised gallbladder shows all the signs of acute inflammation. With experienced surgeons, and patients under the age of 60, mortality is negligible. See also *Cholecystitis, acute emphysematous*

Chronic cholecystitis is chronic inflammation of the gallbladder, often with underlying gallstones. Clinical features are similar to acute cholecystitis, but signs and symptoms are less prominent. Ultrasound of the gallbladder and oral cholecystogram are appropriate investigations, but HIDA scans are not indicated. If symptoms originate from the gallbladder, cholecystectomy is indicated. The pathology of the excised gallbladder is variable, often with minimal signs of chronic inflammation despite a convincing clinical picture and gallstones. (Figure 33 a and b) See also *HIDA scan*

Cholecystitis, acalculous

A condition of inflammation of the gallbladder and bile ducts without gallstones. Causes include starvation and immobility, diabetes mellitus, tumours of the ampulla of Vater, malignant and benign tumours of the bile duct and carcinoma of the gallbladder. Inflammatory lesions of the bile ducts, sclerosing cholangitis, pancreatic disease and, rarely, choledochal cysts may cause cholecystitis. Acalculous cholecystitis also includes adeno-myomatosis of the gallbladder, which is diagnosed on oral cholecystography.

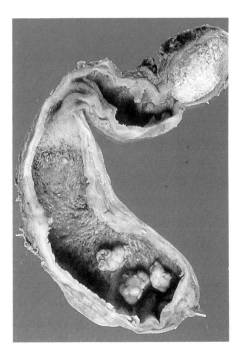

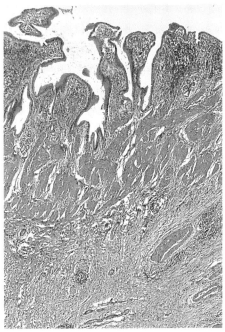

Figure 33a **Cholecystitis.** Chronic cholecystitis and cholelithiasis showing a thickened gallbladder wall with calculi in the fundus and cystic duct.

Figure 33b **Cholecystitis.** The microscopy illustrating a thickened muscular coat of the gallbladder wall and clusters of chronic inflammatory cells throughout. (H.E. x 10).

Cholecystitis

Cholecystitis, acute emphysematous
(*also known as* Gaseous cholecystitis)
This is an infection of the gallbladder
with gas-producing organisms such as
Escherichia coli, *Clostridium welchii*,
or anaerobic *Streptococci*. The clinical
picture is identical to severe acute
cholecystitis but the diagnosis is made
on plain abdominal x-rays, which show a
sharply outlined pear-shaped gas shadow
in the region of the gallbladder. Treatment
is high-dose intravenous antibiotics
combined with cholecystostomy.

Cholecystocolostomy
(*also known as* Colocholecystostomy)
Surgical anastomosis of the gallbladder to
the colon.

Cholecystoenterostomy
see *Cholecystenterostomy*

Cholecystogram
An x-ray of the gallbladder.

Cholecystography (oral)
Oral cholecystography is used for the
diagnosis of gallstones, which are seen as
non-opacified radiolucent areas within
the lumen. Iodine-containing contrast
medium is taken orally, absorbed in the
intestine and transported to the liver. It
is then secreted into the bile ducts and
concentrated in the gallbladder. A fatty
meal is given during cholecystography
to stimulate gallbladder contraction to
verify normal gallbladder functioning. Oral
cholecystography is 98% accurate in the
diagnosis of gallstones, but is unable to
be performed in the presence of
jaundice, when the serum bilirubin is
above 2.0mg per dl. A non-functioning
gallbladder implies pathology provided
the contrast material has been ingested.
Ultrasonography is complementary to oral
cholecystography in the diagnosis of
gallstones, but cholecystography is
superior in diagnosing acalculous
gallbladder disease. (Figure 34) See also
Ultrasonography

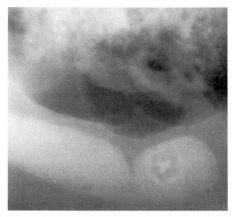

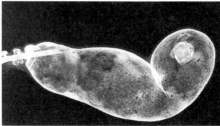

Figure 34 **Cholecystography.** Comparison of
an oral cholecystogram (top) with a double
contrast barium study (bottom) performed
following cholecystectomy. A multi-faceted
gallstone is clearly visible in the fundus of the
gallbladder. (Technique developed by Dr R.
Wilkins and Mrs B. Sandin).

Cholecystokinin (CCK)
(*also known as* Pancreozymin) This is a
polypeptide hormone formed in the
small intestine along with several other
hormones by the cells of the APUD system.
Its main function is to induce contraction
of the gallbladder and pancreatic
secretion. Its exact concentration and
molecular structure are unknown. Under
conditions of gallbladder contraction and
sphincter of Oddi relaxation caused by
CCK, bile is expelled into the duodenum.
See also *Intestinal hormones*

Cholecystostomy

Operative drainage of the gallbladder is performed in acute gallbladder disease if cholecystectomy is inadvisable or technically difficult as, for example, in empyema of the gallbladder. The inflamed gallbladder is not removed but the obstruction is relieved. Antibiotics and the host's natural defences in combination with the cholecystostomy are usually sufficient to relieve symptoms and combat infection and inflammation. An interval cholecystectomy is then performed.

Choledochal

Referring to the common bile duct.

Choledochal cyst

A congenital dilation of the bile ducts, usually affecting the extrahepatic portions. The cyst size varies from two to three cm. up to a capacity of eight litres. The initial clinical presentation is most often in young adults with a triad of symptoms of adominal pain, jaundice and an abdominal mass. Complications in adults are recurrent pancreatitis, portal vein obstruction, portal hypertension and the development of malignancy within the cyst. Investigation by ultrasound, ERCP, or computed tomography of the liver, reveals the bile duct cysts. Surgical excision is the treatment of choice. (Figure 35)

Choledochoenterostomy

Surgical anastomosis of the common bile duct to the intestine, whether duodenum (choledochoduodenostomy), jejunum (choledochojejunostomy), or ileum (choledochoileostomy).

Choledochography

see *Endoscopic retrograde cholangiopancreatography*

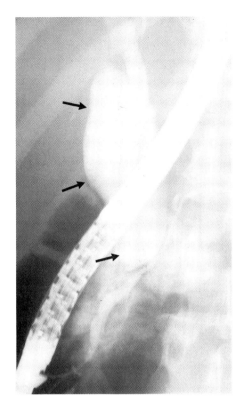

Figure 35 Choledochal cyst. An ERCP showing large filling defect (arrowed) representing a choledochal cyst.

Choledocholithiasis

Multiple or single gallstones situated in the common bile duct. These have usually migrated from the gallbladder so that 10-15% of patients with gallstones in the gallbladder will have stones in the common bile duct. The clinical symptoms are due to intermittent obstruction of the common bile duct leading to jaundice, fever, and right upper quadrant or epigastric pain. Gallstones impacted in the ampulla of Vater may also result in acute pancreatitis.

Ultrasonography, percutaneous transhepatic cholangiography and endoscopic retrograde cholangiopancreatography (ERCP) are useful modes of investigation. Removal of the stones surgically or at ERCP and sphincterotomy, under antibiotic cover, is required. (Figure 36) See also *Cholangitis*

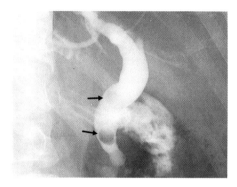

Figure 36 Choledocholithiasis. An ERCP examination which shows two gallstones (arrowed) in the common bile duct.

Choledochoscopy
(*also known as* Choledoscopy)
Examination of the lumen of the intrahepatic and extrahepatic biliary tree performed during surgery to ascertain if the bile ducts are free from gallstones. It is not commonly performed although it decreases the incidence of retained gallstones after cholecystectomy. Flexible fibreoptic choledochoscopes are now available. (Figure 37)

Choledochostomy
Surgical drainage of the common bile duct, which is usually associated with placement of a T-tube catheter.

Choledoscopy
see *Choledochoscopy*

Cholelithiasis
The presence or formation of gallstones. See also *Gallstones*

Cholera
A severe diarrhoeal illness caused by the Gram-negative rod *Vibrio cholerae*. It is endemic in Asia and is transmitted by contaminated food or water (Figure 38). Stool electrolyte losses in cholera were measured as early as 1831 in Scotland and the suggestion for an effective treatment with fluids and electrolytes was made. However, inappropriate suggestions about the pathogenesis hindered rational effective therapy for 120 years.

Pathogenesis Massive fluid loss in the faeces, up to 15-20 litres daily, is caused by the action of the toxin on the intestine. The upper small bowel is particularly vulnerable. The toxin blocks the sodium transport by increasing the adenyl cyclase activity in the intestinal epithelial cell. *Vibrio cholerae* does not invade the mucosal surface. The incubation period is one to five days and unless treatment is commenced, death will follow within 24 hours.

Clinical features Profuse diarrhoea rapidly causes dehydration, the stools being described as ricewater (cloudy, watery and containing mucus but no blood). Cramping abdominal pain and vomiting occur in the initial stage but fever is typically absent.

Treatment Antibiotics, such as tetracycline or chloramphenicol eradicate the organisms from the stool and improve the clinical illness by 50-60%. However,

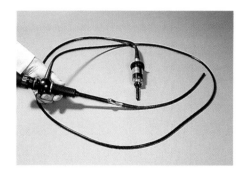

Figure 37 Choledochoscopy. A fibreoptic instrument seen here with flexible tip and manual controls.

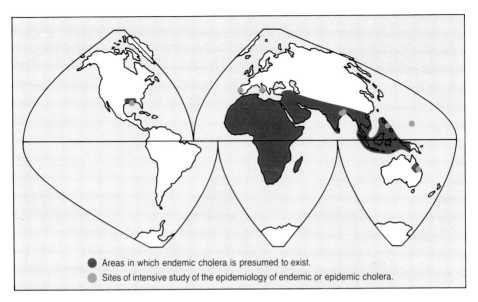

Areas in which endemic cholera is presumed to exist.
Sites of intensive study of the epidemiology of endemic or epidemic cholera.

Figure 38 Cholera. Map illustrating the principle regions of the world affected by cholera.

antibiotics are no substitute for parenteral or enteral fluid replacement, which is the cornerstone of management. The mortality rate is over 50%, but can be reduced to 1% with appropriate measures. The discovery that sugars such as glucose facilitate the absorption of enterally-administered salt and water has transformed the management and outcome in Third World countries.

Cholera (pancreatic)
Profuse watery diarrhoea, hypokalaemia, and achlorhydria, caused by a pancreatic islet-cell tumour or any APUDoma producing VIP (Vasoactive-intestinal peptide).

Choleresis
The production of bile by the liver.

Cholescintigraphy
Radioisotopes have been used to investigate gallbladder disease. It is of most value clinically in acute cholecystitis. Cholescintigraphy involves visualization of the gallbladder by radiolabelled substances injected intravenously and rapidly excreted by the liver, bile ducts, gallbladder, and intestine, within one hour of injection. A normal cholescintogram excludes the diagnosis of acute cholecystitis (Table 7).

Cholestasis
This is obstruction to the outflow of bile caused by pathology either, primarily in the biliary system, or in the liver cells. Clinically this results in jaundice, either obstructive or hepatocellular. The other main category of jaundice due to overproduction of bile pigment from red blood cell destruction (haemolysis) is not strictly cholestatic. There are many causes of cholestasis (Table 8). Pathologically bile pigment is seen in the liver and depending on the cause the changes will commence in the portal tracts (in obstructive jaundice) or in the liver lobules (in hepatocellular jaundice). Besides jaundice clinical symptoms also include pruritis, pale stools and dark urine. Investigation

Cholestasis

Table 7 Uses of cholescintigraphy

Evaluation of suspected cholecystitis
Acute cholecystitis
Chronic cholecystitis
Acalculous cholecystitis
Evaluation of cholestasis
Hepatocellular disease
Bile duct obstruction
Evaluation of the biliary system after surgery or trauma
Bile leak
Biliary-enteric patency after diversionary procedures
Bile-gastric reflux after gastric surgery
Cystic duct remnant after cholecystectomy
Evaluation of biliary anomalies
Choledochal cyst
Caroli's disease
Biliary atresia
Miscellaneous
Correlation with technetium-99m sulphur studies
Correlation with ultrasound study
Liver transplant evaluation
Hepatoma imaging – primary metastases
Liver metastases imaging

with ultrasound or computed tomography will delineate the structure of the intrahepatic and extrahepatic biliary tree. Gallstones in the gallbladder, bile duct, or a pancreatic tumour may be revealed. Percutaneous transhepatic cholangiography and ERCP directly visualize the bile ducts, and are the most definitive investigations in cholestasis. Intrahepatic cholestasis (hepatocellular) occurring in the absence of extrahepatic bile duct obstruction may be due to a late stage of viral hepatitis, drug reactions, primary biliary cirrhosis, or as a manifestation of a malignant disease elsewhere. (Figure 39)

Cholestasis (benign, intrahepatic, recurrent)
(*also known as* Byler's disease) A very rare condition presenting with many separate episodes of cholestasis for which no cause can be found. Symptoms usually begin in childhood and a familial history may be present.

Cholestatic jaundice
see *Jaundice, cholestatic*

Cholesterol
Cholesterol is a sterol which resembles fat and is metabolized widely throughout the body. It is a constituent of cell membrane and various tissues, a precursor for hormone synthesis, and is involved in the production of bile acids. Most cholesterol is synthesized in the liver, the remainder being absorbed from the diet. Elevated serum cholesterol levels which may be genetically based are associated with

Table 8 Causes of cholestasis

Intrahepatic
End-stage cirrhosis
Primary biliary cirrhosis
Drugs
Tumour; metastatic, primary
Acute viral hepatitis
Alcohol
Chronic active hepatitis
Sclerosing cholangitis
Infiltration, for example, Hodgkin's disease, lymphoma
Postoperative
Infection
Pregnancy
Benign recurrent hepatic
Extrahepatic
Stone in the common bile duct
Carcinoma of the pancreas
Stricture of the bile duct, for example, postoperative
Cholangiocarcinoma
Chronic calcific pancreatitis
Carcinoma of the gallbladder
Hydatid cyst
Acute cholecystitis

56

atheroma and its consequences. Normal serum levels are 3.6-7.8 mmol/l (140-300 mg/100 ml). In bile, cholesterol is soluble because of its association with bile salts and phospholipids forming mixed micelles. When the amount of cholesterol in bile increases beyond a certain level it becomes supersaturated, which is an essential factor in gallstone formation. Cholesterol gallstones increase with increasing age and are more common in women. See also *Bile: Gallstones*

Cholesterol gallstones
see *Gallstones, cholesterol*

Cholesterol saturation index
A system for identifying the relative degrees of saturation or supersaturation of bile. Concentrations of cholesterol, bile salts and lecithin are represented each on the three sides of an equilateral triangle. A single point within the triangle may predict cholesterol saturation or supersaturation.

Cholesterolosis of gallbladder
Deposits of cholesterol within submucosal macrophages in the gallbladder. This condition is usually associated with cholesterol gallstones or supersaturated bile, but does not necessarily produce symptoms. The gallbladder mucosa shows multiple yellow flecks and is described as a 'strawberry gallbladder'.

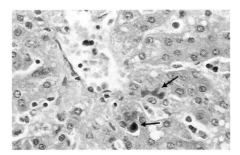

Figure 39 Cholestasis. Bile thrombi in the liver (arrowed) from a patient with drug-induced cholestasis. (HVg x 160).

Cholestyramine
An unpleasant tasting, orally active drug that binds bile acids, preventing their reabsorption in the terminal ileum. It is effective in relieving pruritis in obstructive jaundice or primary biliary cirrhosis and it can be used in patients with extensive terminal ileal disease, for example, Crohn's disease, where bile acid induced diarrhoea may be a problem after small intestinal resection. Cholestyramine also lowers serum cholesterol levels. Side-effects include constipation, nausea and heartburn.

Choluria
The presence of bile in the urine causes it to become dark and is associated with obstructive jaundice. See also *Jaundice*

Chronic
A disease of slow change, usually of long duration. See also *Acute: specific disorders*

Chyle
Opaque milky alkaline fluid, present in lacteals, and consisting of lymph and chylomicrons in a stable emulsion. Chyle is absorbed from the intestine during digestion, and is transported in the lymph to the thoracic duct and from there to the blood.

Chylomicrons
Tiny particles composed mainly of triglyceride (fat) with small amounts of cholesterol, and phospholipid. They are found in intestinal lymphatics after meals, and are an integral part of lipid absorption.

Chylothorax
(*also known as* Chylopleura) The presence of effused chyle in the thoracic cavity.

Chylous ascites
Ascites caused by accumulation of chyle in the peritoneal cavity. Causes of this rare condition include neoplastic,

Chyme

inflammatory, or traumatic conditions usually with obstruction of the thoracic lymph duct.

Chyme
A semiliquid acid collection of material produced by the combined effect of gastric acid, pepsin and motility on food as it is passed into the duodenum.

Chymotrypsin
A proteolytic enzyme produced by the pancreas and secreted in the inactive form chymotrypsinogen. This is converted to chymotrypsin in the intestine by the action of enterokinase. Chymotrypsin hydrolyzes food proteins into peptones, polypeptides and amino acids, by disrupting the peptide linkages between tyrosine and phenylalanine in carboxyl groups.

Cimetidine
A histamine H_2 antagonist which rapidly inhibits both basal and stimulated gastric secretion of acid and reduces pepsin output. It is available orally and intravenously, healing 70-90% of peptic ulcers in six to eight weeks.
Side effects include skin rash, dizziness, reversible confusional states (usually in the elderly), diarrhoea, muscle aches and occasionally gynaecomastia. Cimetidine can prolong the elimination of drugs metabolised by oxidation in the liver. Therefore care must be taken to avoid clinically significant drug interactions, namely those with warfarin, phenytoin, or theophylline. See also H_2 antagonists.

Cirrhosis of the liver
A pathological process involving the entire liver in which there is diffuse fibrosis combined with regenerating nodules. No normal liver architecture remains (Figure 40). It occurs in response to liver-cell injury and persistent inflammation accompanied by fibrosis and compensatory hyperplasia. Although there are many causes the end result is the same.

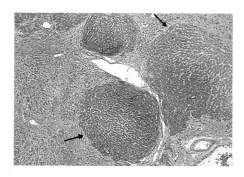

Figure 40 Cirrhosis. Complete destruction of the liver architecture is shown with the formation of regenerative nodules (arrowed) isolated by broad fibrous tracts. (Masson trichrome x 10).

Classification There are two anatomical classifications:
Micronodular Small regenerating uniform nodules are present with thick, regular septa (up to 3 mm diameter).
Macronodular Nodules are of varying size and tend to be larger than micronodular cirrhosis (up to 1 cm diameter).
Causes of cirrhosis The causes are listed in Table 9. In the United Kingdom alcohol is the commonest cause of hepatic cirrhosis but after intensive investigation there remains a group of patients (30%) where no cause is found (*cryptogenic cirrhosis*). Rarely, cirrhosis may be attributable to persistent passive liver congestion (*cardiac cirrhosis*) or due to biliary cholestasis (*biliary cirrhosis*).
Clinical features Cirrhosis results in liver cell failure and portal hypertension. The patient who is well-compensated may have no symptoms. However, most patients complain of fatigue, minor weight loss or reduced libido. Clinical signs include palmar erythema, leuconychia, finger clubbing, spider naevae and jaundice. Occasionally axillary hair loss, gynaecomastia and testicular atrophy may occur. Abdominal examination often shows splenomegaly, which indicates

Table 9 Causes of cirrhosis

Alcohol

Hepatitis B, non-A, non-B

Metabolic, for example, Wilson's disease,

Haemochromatosis, alpha-1-antitrypsin deficiency

Hepatic vein occlusion, for example, Budd-Chiari syndrome

Persistent bile duct obstruction

Lupoid hepatitis and primary biliary cirrhosis

Drugs, for example, Methotrexate

Indian childhood cirrhosis

Cryptogenic infections

portal hypertension, or ascites. Depending on the cause of cirrhosis, the liver may be enlarged or reduced in size. Bacterial infections, tuberculosis, alterations of carbohydrate metabolism, osteomalacia and osteoporosis, all occur more frequently in patients with liver cirrhosis.

Investigations should be directed towards the four main areas referred to in Table 10.

Treatment is dependent on the underlying condition. An adequate diet and avoidance of alcohol are sensible precautions. The diet should include 1gm protein/kg bodyweight, unless the patient is cachetic or encephalopathic. There is no therapeutic benefit in avoiding butter, fats, eggs, milk, or chocolate. If ascites or portal hypertension is present, sodium restriction combined with carefully monitored diuresis is appropriate. In lupoid hepatitis, corticosteroids reduce hepatic inflammation, and prolong survival. In haemochromatosis, venesection followed by desferrioxamine should be employed, while in Wilson's disease the early use of the copper chelating drug penicillamine is essential. Portal hypertension frequently results from liver cirrhosis. See also *Portal hypertension*

Prognosis The prognostic signs and symptoms are referred to in Table 11.

Cirrhosis types

Alcoholic cirrhosis (also known as Laennec's cirrhosis) Postulated causes are nutritional deficiency, direct toxic effect of alcohol, toxic metabolites of alcohol, for example, acetaldehyde. Mallory's hyaline is a useful diagnostic histologic feature.

Biliary cirrhosis Caused by long-standing obstruction of or damage to the biliary system and characterized by jaundice, steatorrhoea, liver and spleen enlargement. See also *Primary biliary cirrhosis: Secondary biliary cirrhosis*

Cardiac cirrhosis Caused by congestive heart failure. Associated with scarring around the central veins of the hepatic lobules.

Table 10 Investigations for Cirrhosis

Objective	Investigation
Confirm diagnosis	Liver biopsy (if possible)
Find underlying cause	Hepatitis B serology Autoantibody tests Serum ferritin
Assess liver cell function	Liver function tests Serum albumin Coagulation profile
Assess portasystemic collateral circulation	Barium swallow Gastroscopy

Table 11 Signs and symptoms indicating poor prognosis in cirrhosis

Jaundice

Ascites

Small, shrunken liver

Lack of significant treatment response in one month

Persistent hypotension

Low serum albumin (< 25gm/l)

Hyponatraemia (Na < 120mequv/l) without diuretics

Persistently prolonged prothrombin time

Variceal bleeding

Cirrhosis

Indian childhood cirrhosis A rare condition of unknown aetiology affecting young children of Indian families. Sex incidence is equal, the disorder presenting in the first few years of life with failure to thrive, hepatomegaly and low grade pyrexia. Later, portal hypertension develops. Liver histology shows severe liver cell damage, Mallory's hyaline bodies and micronodular cirrhosis. There is a prominent polymorph infiltration but no associated fat. High copper levels are found within the liver, necessitating the exclusion of Wilson's disease. Unfortunately, death is almost inevitable.

Postnecrotic cirrhosis A condition which follows a submassive necrosis of the liver. Causes are toxic or viral hepatitis. See also *Acute yellow atrophy*

Primary biliary cirrhosis A condition of developing liver cirrhosis found most commonly in middle-aged women in which there are immunological features such as positive antimitochondrial antibodies. These antibodies are a marker of disease rather than an aetiological agent.

Pathological features are gradual destruction of medium and small bile ducts accompanied by inflammation, granulomas and dissection of the liver structure. Raised levels of hepatic copper are present.

Clinical manifestations are pruritus, jaundice, hypercholesterolaemia, xanthelasma and later hepato-splenomegaly.

Treatment is supportive with replacement of fat soluble vitamins, together with calcium. There is no evidence that penicillamine is useful in treating this condition.

Prognosis Good prognostic features are: bilirubin less than 30 per 100 ml, granulomas on liver biopsy, absence of hepatosplenomegaly.

Secondary biliary cirrhosis is caused by chronic bile obstruction due to congenital atresia or stricture.

Clonorchiasis

A liver fluke infestation occurring in the Far East, caused by ingestion of uncooked or partially cooked infected fish. The cysts are ingested and larvae develop in the duodenum and eventually reach the bile ducts. Clinical symptoms include cholangitis and hepatomegaly. Laboratory investigations reveal eosinophilia and raised serum alkaline phosphatase of liver origin. The diagnosis is made on discovering cysts in the faeces, and treatment with praziquantel should be started.

Clostridium botulinum

This is the bacterium (formerly called *Bacillus botulinus*) causing botulism in man and some animals. *Clostridium botulinum* is an anaerobic, spore-forming, Gram-positive rod, which produces a powerful exotoxin resistance to proteolytic digestion. It may be classified into various types such as A, B, C alpha and beta, D, and E on the basis of the immunological specificity of the toxin. See also *Botulism*

Clubbing of the fingers

Excess production of soft tissue around the ends of the fingers (or toes) causes loss of the normal angle between the nail beds and fingers. This results in increased movement of the nail, corroborating the clinical sign. There are many causes of clubbing but important gastroenterological causes are Crohn's disease, coeliac disease, cystic fibrosis of the pancreas and chronic cholestatic liver disease. (Figure 41)

Cobalamin absorption
see *Vitamin B$_{12}$ absorption*

Codeine phosphate

An opiate-based drug which reduces colonic motility and is useful in controlling diarrhoea.

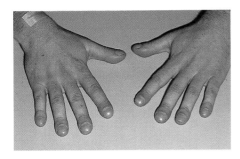

Figure 41 Clubbing of the fingers.

Coeliac
Relating to the abdominal region.

Coeliac artery
A large vessel from the abdominal aorta arising at the level of the twelfth thoracic vertebrae and supplying three major branches, namely the splenic, left gastric and hepatic arteries. (Figure 42)

Coeliac compression syndrome
(*also known as* Median arcuate ligament syndrome) This syndrome consists of recurrent abdominal pain associated with a narrowing of the coeliac artery. Most patients are women complaining of epigastric pain and infrequently of nausea and vomiting. On examination, an abdominal bruit is present. Coeliac artery angiography confirms the diagnosis by showing narrowing of the coeliac axis near its origin. Results of surgery are unpredictable.

Coeliac disease
(*also known as* Coeliac sprue: Gluten sensitive enteropathy: Non-tropical sprue) A disorder affecting the small intestine (mainly jejunum and duodenum) due to sensitivity of the intestine to a protein, gliadin, which is part of the gluten fraction of wheat and rye. Malabsorption of all nutrients may occur, together with non-specific but typical small bowel biopsy appearances affecting the mucosa but sparing submucosa, muscularis mucosa

and serosa. Rapid clinical improvement occurs when gluten is withdrawn from the diet, while histological changes should revert to normal within three to six months. This condition affects 0.03% to 0.1% of the population. However, in the West of Ireland, the incidence is as high as one in 300. The pathology in untreated coeliac patients reveals flattened villi, elongated crypts, and increased intraepithelial lymphocyte counts. Mucosal enzymes such as disaccharidases are reduced.

Genetic factors may influence the disorder because approximately 80% of patients have the HLA configuration HLA-B8, compared with 20% of the normal adult population. Cell-mediated immunity may affect the pathogenesis and it has been suggested that T lymphocytes in the lamina propria may produce lymphokines in response to gluten.

Clinical symptoms The severity of symptoms depends upon the extent of the disease. Malabsorption is prominent with stunted growth in children, diarrhoea, steatorrhoea, flatulence, weight loss and weakness. A typical stool is large, greasy, pale and offensive. Anaemia and its symptoms are not uncommon, due to nutritional deficiencies, for example, impaired iron and folate absorption from the proximal intestine.

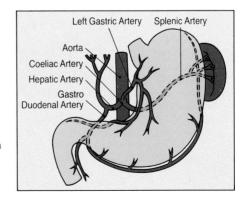

Figure 42 Coeliac artery.

Coeliac disease

Osteomalacia and osteoporosis may develop with the disturbance of calcium transport and vitamin D absorption. Physical examination findings vary widely. Evidence of anaemia, cachexia, finger clubbing, oedema, leukonychia, glossitis, angular cheilosis, and hypocalcaemia, indicate extensive severe disease.

Laboratory investigations Intestinal biopsy is the gold standard for diagnosis. A peroral biopsy capsule is positioned fluoroscopically and 'fired' under suction with a syringe. All other investigations are ancillary but useful in assessing the extent of the disease. Faecal fat estimations are elevated, anaemia is usually due to folate or iron deficiency, while hypocalcaemia is caused by malabsorption of calcium and vitamin D. The xylose absorption test is a sensitive test for coeliac disease. Radiology of the small bowel reveals a distorted mucosal fold pattern, flocculation of barium and dilated small bowel loops. (Figure 43)

Treatment This is removal of gluten from the diet. In practice this is difficult. Wheat products are in many processed foods, for example, some ice-creams, sauces, salad dressing and many canned foods. Rice, soybean and cornflour are not toxic, but oats should probably be eliminated from the diet. Coeliac Societies disseminate up-to-date information about specific foods and are a useful way of patients sharing ideas, recipes and problems. Some patients tolerate small amounts of gluten, while others are exquisitely sensitive to dietary indiscretions. Initially, anaemia and hypocalcaemia require specific parenteral therapy, followed later by oral therapy. Vitamins A, B, C and E should be given as a multivitamin preparation.

Complications The development of lymphoma is a rare, but real risk, occurring in 5% of coeliac patients. Other internal carcinomas, in particular oesophageal carcinoma are more common. Small bowel stricturing and ulceration are very rare and a disputed complication in the absence of associated malignancy. In such

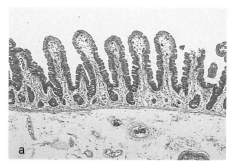

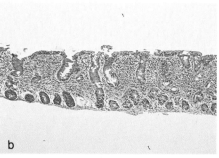

Figure 43 Coeliac disease. Comparison of normal jejunal mucosa (a) with flat mucosa (b) from a case of coeliac disease. (H.E. x 25).

cases the disease is often refractory to treatment of withdrawal of gluten and then corticosteroids are a useful adjunct. See also *Gluten enteropathy*

Coeliac sprue
see *Coeliac disease*

Colectomy
Surgical removal of part or all of the colon. Total colectomy requires the formation of an ileostomy or ileorectal pouch and is undertaken in patients with fulminating ulcerative colitis. Right hemicolectomy is performed for patients with right-sided colon disease, for example, cancer, Crohn's disease or angiodysplasia. Left hemicolectomy is undertaken in patients with left-sided lesions such as cancer, ischaemia, or severe complicated diverticular disease.

Colic

The description given to severe abdominal pain which often arises from distension or obstruction of the intestine. The pain fluctuates, arriving in waves either seconds or minutes apart. The presence of colic suggests partial or complete intestinal obstruction, or the development of severe constipation. In infants, colic may occur associated with feeding and is more common in breast-fed babies. Small intestinal colic is felt in the upper abdomen, while colonic colic is experienced below the umbilicus. Many different organs may be responsible for colic, for example, biliary colic from bile ducts, usually associated with gallstones, or pancreatic colic from pancreatic stones obstructing the pancreatic duct.

Colitis

An inflammatory change within the colon with many different causes, such as radiation, infection, ischaemia, Crohn's colitis and ulcerative colitis. Histological changes depend on the cause of the colitis. Inflammation limited to the mucosa with crypt abscesses occurs in ulcerative colitis, while in Crohn's colitis, focal full thickness bowel inflammation is observed with granulomas in about 60% of cases.

Clinical symptoms include abdominal pain, diarrhoea with blood mucus, and perhaps pus.

Treatment of the colitis depends on the cause. Ulcerative colitis and Crohn's colitis are treated with sulphasalazine and corticosteroids. Severe fulminating colitis may require colectomy. Amoebic colitis due to *Entamoeba histolytica* is treated with amoebicidal drugs. Pseudomembranous colitis due to *Clostridium difficile* is treated with metronidazole or vancomycin. See also *Amoebic colitis: Collagenous colitis: Crohn's disease: Ischaemic colitis: Pseudomembranous colitis: Radiation colitis: Ulcerative colitis*

Collagenous colitis

A rare condition of unknown aetiology recently described, in which there is a thick collagen band greater than 10 microns in the subepithelial region of the colonic mucosa. The small bowel is not involved. Symptoms include watery diarrhoea (without blood) and cramping abdominal pain. The disorder has a predilection for middle-aged and elderly women, but no specific therapy has been found to provide reliable control of symptoms. There appears to be no complication from this disease apart from the discomfort and inconvenience of symptoms.

Collagenous sprue

An uncommon disorder of unknown cause with a poor prognosis affecting only the small bowel. There is a dense subepithelial collagen band which does not respond to a gluten-free diet or corticosteroids. No relationship with collagenous colitis has been found.

Collateral veins, abdominal wall

These veins develop with increasing resistance to blood flow within the portal veins when portal pressure rises above 10 mmHg. Therefore, portal blood is diverted into the systemic veins. They are associated with oesophageal varices, haemorrhoids and a caput medusae. Cirrhosis of the liver is the most common cause.

Colocholecystostomy

see *Cholecystocolostomy*

Coloenteric fistula

A fistula or communication between the colon and the small intestine which may occur as a complication of a diverticular abscess which ruptures into the small intestine. Frequently these fistulas are asymptomatic but if bacterial overgrowth occurs, diarrhoea and steatorrhoea may result.

Coloenteritis

see *Enterocolitis*

Colon

The large intestine is divided into five parts; caecum, ascending, transverse, descending and sigmoid colon. Its main functions are to carry the waste products of digestion to the rectum for expulsion from the body (defaecation) and to absorb fluids and electrolytes from the undigested material. Peristalsis forces faeces towards the rectum prior to defaecation. The colon decreases in width from the caecum to anus and has both circular and longitudinal muscle fibres. The latter are gathered into three bands, the taeniae coli. The colon is well supplied with arteries, veins and lymphatics, the main blood supply coming from the superior and inferior mesenteric arteries. Ileal contents reach the colon via the ileocaecal valve which opens into the caecum or first part of the colon, discharging its contents. The colon can be directly visualized at colonoscopy or seen radiographically on plain films of the abdomen or at barium enema. (Figure 44)

Giant colon and pelvic colon are known as megacolon and sigmoid colon respectively and may be referred to under these headings. Lead-pipe colon is a descriptive radiological term for a colon which has become featureless and shortened following chronic inflammation, usually

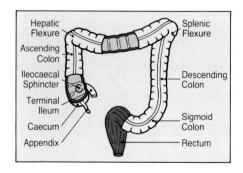

Figure 44 Colon.

secondary to ulcerative colitis or Crohn's colitis.

Colon, cathartic

see *Laxative abuse*

Colonic carcinoma

Colonic carcinoma is one of the most common neoplasms in the Western world. If rectal carcinoma is included, it is second only to carcinoma of the lung. The incidence of colonic carcinoma increases with age as the mean age for presentation is between 60 and 70 years. It occasionally occurs in young people and this is more common in low prevalence areas. The sex incidence is approximately equal, which is in contrast to rectal carcinoma, which is more common in men.

Causes The cause of colonic carcinoma is not known, though certain conditions predispose to its development. These conditions include inherited disorders such as familial polyposis coli and Gardner's syndrome. There is a four-fold increase of colonic carcinoma amongst relatives of patients with carcinoma and in patients with long-standing extensive ulcerative colitis. The risk can reach as high as 30% after 30 years of the disease. However, it is the adenomatous polyp which is the most important predisposing factor from the screening point of view. It is likely that all colonic carcinomas commence as benign adenomatous polyps. Such a polyp is deemed a cancer when its dysplastic epithelium penetrates the muscularis mucosae into the polyp stalk.

Aetiology Environmental factors play a role in the aetiology of colonic carcinoma as it is virtually unknown in most of the Third World population. These peoples have bulkier stools and more frequent bowel movements than in the West. There is less time for carcinogens to reside in the colon. Altered bacterial flora, their metabolites and secondary bile acids have also been implicated. Finally, the incidence of colonic carcinoma is more common in populations who consume large amounts of dietary fat but have a low content of cereal fibre.

Types The vast majority of colonic carcinomas are adenocarcinomas. Nearly 50% occur in the recto-sigmoid area, 25% in the sigmoid colon, and the remainder are equally distributed between the caecum, ascending colon, transverse colon and descending colon. The tumour is spread by local invasion and distant dissemination in the blood and lymphatics. Approximately 5% of patients have more than one colonic carcinoma and the incidence of synchronous cancers increases with the number of adenomas.

Clinical features Typical presentation of colonic carcinoma is a change in bowel habit with bleeding. Abdominal pain and weight loss are common. Iron deficiency anaemia may be the sole manifestation with occult right-sided colonic tumours. Rectal bleeding is perhaps the most useful symptom diagnostically. Most patients with colonic carcinoma will require a barium enema, although those with intestinal obstruction may need urgent surgery. Colonoscopy and biopsy are also an important part of the diagnostic process.

The majority of colonic carcinomas are small, circumscribed and ulcerated with raised edges. Fungating polypoid tumours are less common and predominate in the caecum. Diffusely infiltrating carcinomas akin to a gastric 'linitis plastica' are rare. Residual benign adenomatous tissue can be found in approximately 15% of cases, supporting the polyp-cancer sequence.

Prognosis depends on the histological grade of the tumour and its spread which is commonly classified according to Dukes' staging. In Dukes' A stage, the tumour is confined to the bowel wall and 5-year survival approaches 90%. Malignant polyps with the tumour limited to the stalk are Dukes' A stage and polypectomy is adequate therapy. In Dukes' B lesions, tumour growth is beyond the muscularis propria and 5-year survival is approximately 70%. When lymph nodes

are involved, it is a Dukes' stage C lesion. Prognosis then depends on the number and site of the lymph nodes involved, but average 5-year survivals are below 30%.

Colonoscope

A long flexible fibreoptic instrument whose tip can be moved in all directions by means of control wheels at the head. The entire colon may be visualized directly, biopsies obtained, polyps removed, and bleeding points such as angiodysplasias diathermied. (Figure 45)

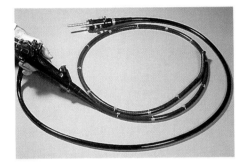

Figure 45 Colonoscope. A 1.5m. flexible instrument used for visualizing the colon. The tip may be manipulated in all directions using the control wheels.

Colonoscopy

In this procedure the colonoscope is used to visualize the entire colon. The instrument is passed via the rectum through the sigmoid, descending, transverse and ascending colon to the caecum. Colonic preparation is important to obtain a good view and biopsies may be taken of abnormal areas while polyps can be snared, diathermied and retrieved. Diathermy may be used for angiodysplasia of the caecum or ascending colon. The procedure requires sedation and analgesia to relieve discomfort. Indications for colonoscopy are diagnosis of suspected colonic cancer, colitis, strictures, colonic ischaemia or angiodysplasia. It is the best, safest method of removing colonic polyps, 5% of which may be cancerous, depending on the size of the polyp. However, colonoscopy is a difficult technique to master and complications include perforation (0.2-0.4%), haemorrhage, explosion (when using diathermy combined with oral mannitol preparation), and infection. See also *Electrocautery*

Colostomy

A surgical procedure where a loop of the colon is brought up through the anterior abdominal wall, and opened so that the contents of the intestine are drained from the stoma into a disposable bag on the abdomen. A colostomy can be performed at any site and may be temporary or permanent. Indications for colostomy include extensive obstructing malignancy of the rectum or sigmoid colon (which requires a permanent colostomy), colonic obstruction from any cause, or extensive rectal Crohn's disease. Complications of colostomy are stoma necrosis, prolapse and stenosis. Abscess formation, fistulae and skin erosions may also occur and initial careful observation is essential in preventing many early colostomy problems. (Figure 46)

Colovesical fistula

A fistula occurring between the sigmoid colon and the posterior wall of the bladder. It occurs uncommonly with diverticulitis when the patient presents with recurrent urinary infections, pneumaturia and faecaluria. See also *Fistula*

Coma, hepatic

Hepatic coma accompanies grade 4 and 5 hepatic encephalopathy and is associated with typical electroencephalographic (EEG) changes, that is, slowing of the alpha rhythm to four cycles/second. The cause of coma is multifactorial including ammonia toxicity, excess nitrogen absorption and possible defects in the blood-brain barrier. See also *Hepatic encephalopathy*

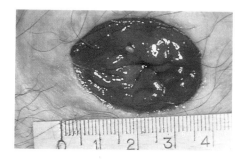

Figure 46 Colostomy. Sigmoid colostomy.

Combined immunodeficiency disease
see *Immunodeficiency disease, combined*

Common bile duct
see *Bile duct*

Common variable immunodeficiency, and gastrointestinal disorders

A rare combination of disorders with B cell and, occasionally, T cell dysfunction. Serum immunoglobulin levels are low and diarrhoea and malabsorption due to *Giardia lamblia* infections commonly result. Nodular lymphoid hyperplasia is also a feature in the small bowel best seen during intestinal radiology.

Computed tomography scanning

(*also known as* Computed(terized) axial tomography scanning: CT scan) This is a radiological technique for the examination of soft tissues. The x-ray scanner beam records 'slices' of the body which are processed by a computer to give cross-sectional images of any part of the body including head, chest, abdomen and pelvis. In gastroenterology this technique is of particular value in imaging the abdomen and pelvis where liver metastatic disease, pancreatic neoplasms and abdominal abscesses may be visualized. Lymphoma with extraperitoneal involvement, gallstones and choledocholithiasis accompanied by dilation of the intrahepatic, common hepatic and common bile ducts are also well seen. There are many advantages with CT scanning which can differentiate small density differences between substances and can accurately distinguish between tissues containing varying amounts of water, blood, fat, bone, gas, or calcium. The investigation is noninvasive, rapid and safe; the radiation dose is usually less than a barium enema. Computed tomography equipment is not difficult to operate, but is expensive to buy, service and maintain. The films are best interpreted by radiologists with a special interest in CT scanning necessitating close liason between gastroenterologist and radiologist.

Congenital hepatic fibrosis
see *Hepatic fibrosis*

Constipation
The passage of hard stool, associated with infrequent and difficult defaecation. This may be due to a low fibre diet, poor colonic motility or colonic denervation. It is more common in the elderly, where careful drug prescribing is particularly important. It may herald organic disease particularly if of recent onset. Local colonic pathology or a more generalized condition such as hypothyroidism or hypercalcaemia may be responsible. Constipation is not a diagnosis but a symptom which should warrant careful, thorough medical evaluation of the patient.

Coprophagia
Coprophagy, or the ingestion of faeces.

Coproporphyria
A rare hereditary condition due to a defect in an enzyme in the porphyrin pathway. Symptoms are unusual but when they do occur take the form of abdominal pain and neuropsychiatric manifestations. There is excess excretion of coproporphyrin in the faeces. See also *Porphyria*

Coprostasis
Faecal impaction.

Corticosteroids
Any steroid hormone produced by the adrenal cortex. There are two main subgroups, excluding androgenic steroids.
Mineralocorticoids, for example, aldosterone, which regulates salt and water balance.
Glucocorticoids, for example, an integral part of hydrocortisone, which is the regulation of cell metabolism. Corticosteroids (glucocorticoids) are used for the treatment of inflammatory bowel disease and chronic active hepatitis. See also *Prednisolone: Steroids*

Courvoisier's law (sign)
(Ludwig Georg Courvoisier, Swiss surgeon, 1843-1918)
This states that an enlarged gallbladder in the presence of obstructive jaundice is likely to be caused by conditions other than gallstones.

Crigler-Najjar syndrome
(John Fielding Crigler Jr, U.S. physician, born 1919: Victor Assad Najjar, Lebanese-born U.S. paediatrician, born 1914)
A severe familial form of non-haemolytic jaundice in which there is a grossly raised unconjugated bilirubin level. This rare condition is due to deficiency of

Table 12 Causes of constipation

Colonic disease: tumours, diverticular disease, muscle or nervous disorders

Small intestinal disease: obstruction

Rectal disease: fissures, fistula, ulcers, Hirschsprung's disease

Metabolic: hyperthyroidism, lead poisoning, hypercalcaemia, depression

Drugs: opiates and related drugs, anticholinergic preparations, antacids antiparkinsonian drugs, tricyclic antidepressants, clonidine HCl

Faulty bowel habits

conjugating enzyme in the liver. See also *Hyperbilirubinaemia*

Crohn's disease
(Burrill Bernard Crohn, U.S. physician, born 1884)
Crohn's disease is a disorder of unknown aetiology which can affect any part of the gastrointestinal tract from mouth to anus. Inflammation is the hallmark of this disease with predilection for the terminal ileum, colon and anus. Many different aetiological factors have been examined but no infectious agent has yet been isolated. The disorder tends to occur in families but not in spouses which has prompted investigation into immuno-logical factors. There is increased anergy in Crohn's disease with reduced T lymphocytes in serum and excess B cells in the affected mucosa.
Crohn's disease usually affects young adults although it may begin in childhood or in elderly patients. Certain races, for example, Jews and Europeans, have a high prevalence, but blacks have a low prevalence.

Pathology Crohn's disease involving the intestine is typically a disease of segmental areas of colon or small intestine. It is a disease of the full thickness of the bowel wall manifest by development of fistulas and deep fissures. Stricturing of the intestine is common. Microscopically transmural inflammation, submucosal fibrosis, fissuring ulceration and discrete granulomas occur (Figure 47 a b and c).

Clinical features Abdominal pain occurs in 95% of patients, diarrhoea in 92%, weight loss in 85%, and fever in 56%. These are the most common symptoms of Crohn's disease. In Britain there is a tendency for patients to have colonic involvement alone which occurs in 30-50% of patients. Lower gastrointestinal bleeding is also common while anal fissures and abscesses occur in one third of patients, presenting a real therapeutic challenge. Diarrhoea may be aggravated by fat malabsorption, bile salt deconjugation,

bacterial overgrowth and secondary lactose intolerance. Extra-colonic features occur in one quarter of patients and are listed in Table 13.

Investigation (diagnostic) A histological diagnosis is essential and when rectal or endoscopic biopsies fail to reach diseased sites surgery may be necessary to obtain tissue. Endoscopy also helps delineate the extent of the disease and monitor its progress. Anal tags, fistulas, abscesses and fissures are more common in colonic disease. The barium enema may show skip lesions with stricturing. The rectum is often spared which is in contrast to ulcerative

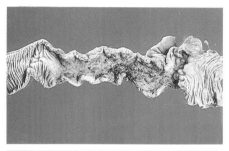

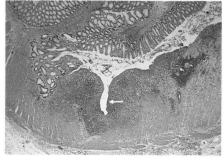

Figure 47a Crohn's disease. Crohn's disease of the terminal ileum with ulceration and a stricture. The normal caecum is seen on the right.

Figure 47b Crohn's disease. In this section of Crohn's disease there is fissuring ulceration, transmural inflammation and surviving mildly inflamed mucosa. (H.E. x 8).

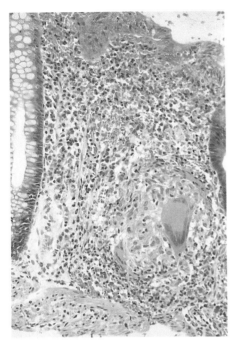

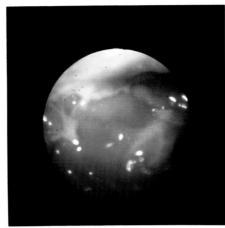

Figure 47c Crohn's disease. A giant cell granuloma in the colonic mucosa. (H.E. x 63).
Figure 47d Crohn's disease. Endoscopic view of a patient with Crohn's disease. Note the ulcerated areas associated with nodularity.

colitis. Reflux of contrast material into the terminal ileum may show nodularity, irregularity and narrowing. Barium follow-through or small bowel enema outlines the pattern of small intestinal involvement. (Figure 47d and e)

Investigation (ancillary) Anaemia, raised ESR, and acute phase proteins such as C-reactive protein (CRP) occur. Vitamin B_{12} deficiency is rare except when there has been a surgical resection of the terminal ileum. The serum proteins and albumin are low in extensive disease. Stool culture and microscopy should always be performed to exclude infection, and amoebic complement fixation test help to exclude amoebiasis.

Complications These include intestinal obstruction, fistula formation, perforation, bleeding, and the development of malignancy. Colonic cancer is three times more frequent in patients with Crohn's disease compared with the general population. Systemic complications include spondylitis, sacroiliitis, arthritis, iritis, episcleritis, erythema nodosum and pyoderma gangrenosum. Liver complications are rare but sclerosing cholangitis may occasionally occur. Kidney stones, particularly oxalate stones, may also be associated with Crohn's disease. Thromboses are described in patients with inflammatory bowel disease and are associated with a hypercoagulable state.

Management Nutritional status is extremely important in the management of patients with Crohn's disease, and diets high in protein and calories are to be recommended. Elemental diets have been shown to be effective management for acute flare-ups, especially in small bowel disease. Drugs do not cure Crohn's disease but serve to improve and control the disorder. Some fortunate patients (10-15%) may have long periods of time with no symptoms. However, most require prolonged treatment to suppress disease

Crohn's disease

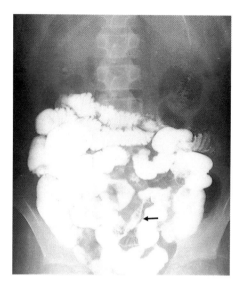

Figure 47e Crohn's disease. Barium follow-through examination showing a stricture in the ileum (arrowed) in a patient with confirmed Crohn's disease.

activity. Prednisolone is effective for suppressing symptoms in exacerbations of disease, especially when ileocaecal, but has no convincing effect on long-term prognosis. Combination treatment with azathioprine has a steroid-sparing effect. Sulfasalazine is most effective in previously untreated patients and may be useful for preventing relapses. However, it

Table 13 Extra-colonic features of Crohn's disease

Fever	50%
Arthritis	25%
Renal stones (oxalate)	20%
Spondylitis	10%
Iritis, episcleritis	7%
Erythema nodosum	5%
Pyoderma gangrenosum	1%
Thomboses	1%
Sclerosing cholangitis	less than 1%

is less effective in Crohn's disease than in ulcerative colitis. Metronidazole has been shown to be equally effective as sulfasalazine in colonic disease. However, peripheral neuropathy occurring in some patients with long term therapy limits its usefulness. Azathioprine used alone is of no benefit. Surgery should be considered when there is intestinal obstruction, fistula formation or evidence of a persistent inflammatory mass. Excision of the diseased bowel is recommended rather than simple removal of fistulous tracts. Bypass surgery with temporary colostomy or ileostomy may be required for severe anal Crohn's disease.

Cromoglycate, for ulcerative colitis
Cromoglycate stabilizes mast cell membranes preventing release of histamine, heparin and serotonin. Initial trials suggested some benefit in ulcerative colitis. However, it has now been established that it is no more effective than placebo and significantly less effective than salazopyrine. It is therefore not recommended for use in ulcerative colitis.

Cronkhite-Canada syndrome
see *Canada-Cronkhite syndrome*

CRST syndrome
Indicates the initial letters of Calcinosis, Raynaud's phenomenon, Sclerodactyly and Telangiectasia, with or without oesophageal motility disorders. When scleroderma is associated with this syndrome the prognosis is improved. CRST may also be found with primary biliary cirrhosis.

Cryptosporidium
A protozoa recognized over the last ten years as a cause of diarrhoea in man. Most patients have some form of immune paresis and when occurring in AIDS patients produce profuse watery diarrhoea which is difficult to treat. Fluid and electrolyte replacement is the main form of therapy.

Crypts of Lieberkühn
(Johannes Nathaniel Lieberkühn, German anatomist, 1711-1756)
Crypts opening on to the mucosa of the large intestine conveying material from the intestinal glands to the surface.

Curling's ulcer
(Thomas Blizard Curling, English physician, 1811-1888)
Acute, multiple, small, superficial gastric erosions or ulcers found in patients with severe burns.

Cushing's ulcer
(Harvey William Cushing, U.S. neurosurgeon, 1869-1939)
Acute ulcers found in the oesophagus, stomach and duodenum which are deeper than Curling's ulcers and may therefore perforate. They are associated with central nervous system trauma or surgery.

Cyclic vomiting
Recurrent episodes of severe vomiting beginning in childhood for which no obvious cause can be found. Attacks may be associated with headache and abdominal pain but between attacks the patient is well. Careful assessment to exclude conditions such as malrotation of the gut or an intracranial tumour is essential. Most patients recover spontaneously, but the cause is unknown.

Cyproheptadine
A serotonin antagonist used to control flushing in carcinoid syndrome with hepatic metastases. It is an orally active drug superior to methysergide which may produce retroperitoneal fibrosis.

Cystadenocarcinoma, pancreatic
A cystic malignant epithelial tumour of the pancreas probably derived from ductular epithelium. It is commonest in middle-age and there is a female preponderance. The tumours range from 5 cms up to 30 cms and occur mostly in the body or tail. These tumours, if completely resected, have a good prognosis.

Table 14 Differential diagnosis: Ulcerative colitis and Crohn's disease

Features	Ulcerative colitis	Crohn's disease
Clinical	Bloody stool usual	Bloody stool less common
Anal lesions	Common	Commoner than ulcerative colitis
Rectal examination	Oedema	Rigid, nodular
Sigmoidoscopy	Bleeding; friable; oedema; no vascular pattern	Purulent, nodular, bleeding
Barium enema	Continuous involvement; shortened colon; predominantly left-sided; associated spasm and pseudo-polyps; strictures rare; dilated ileum	Skip lesions; mainly right-sided; intramural fissures; pseudo-diverticula; strictures common; normal ileum
Cancer	Frequent	Very slight increase
Pathology	Superficial crypt abscesses; goblet cell depletion	Oedema; granulomas; lymphoid hyperplasia; transverse fissures

Cystadenoma, pancreatic

This is a rare benign tumour of the pancreas arising from ductular epithelium. It is more common in women than in men and is mostly sited in the tail. Two forms exist, one is microcystic and the epithelium rich in glycogen. In the other pattern there are large locules lined by mucinous epithelium. This type is premalignant and must be completely excised. A pathological spectrum exists between this pattern and an obvious cystadenocarcinoma.

Cystic duct

The duct which drains bile from the gallbladder into the common hepatic duct. See also *Bile ducts*

Cystic fibrosis of pancreas

Cystic fibrosis is an inherited autosomal recessive disorder affecting children and adolescents. Homozygotes have the disease while heterozygotes are normal. The gene frequency in the population in the United Kingdom is 1 in 25. In cystic fibrosis, abnormalities of all exocrine glands occur.

Clinical features vary from meconium ileus at birth to development of recurrent respiratory infections in childhood. Progressive loss of exocrine pancreatic function occurs in the majority of patients, requiring pancreatic extract supplementation. Diagnosis should be suspected in children who have loose stools and fail to thrive despite good appetites. A sweat test with high sodium concentrations is diagnostic of cystic fibrosis.

Management Control of pulmonary infections with regular physiotherapy, postural drainage, and appropriate, early use of antibiotics is important. Malabsorption is treated with pancreatic supplements. Despite significant progress in the last ten years, life expectancy is still significantly shortened. See also *Fibrosis*

Cysticercosis

A tapeworm infestation acquired by eating partially cooked or raw pork infected with the eggs of *Taenia solium*. The adult worm does not often cause symptoms, but if the eggs penetrate the intestinal wall then cysticercosis may develop with muscle aches and pains, headache, and cerebral symptoms. Diagnosis of cysticercosis depends on excision and histology of the lesion. Worm infestations are diagnosed by finding gravid proglottides in the stool.

Cysts

see *specific types including Choledochal, Hydatid (multilocular)*

Cytomegalovirus infection (CMV)

Cytomegalovirus infection is transmitted by close contact or by congenital infection. It is capable of inducing immunoparesis in susceptible individuals. Cytomegalovirus infection is also an important cause of hepatitis, producing fever and lymphadenopathy. The diagnosis is made by finding raised IgM anti CMV-antibodies in the serum or from culture of the virus from urine or saliva. It is, however, mainly a disease of the immunocompromised rather than a primary pathogen.